Heal From Narcissistic Abuse by Healing Your Inner Child

Break the Pattern of Narcissistic Relationships and Get the Love You Deserve by Healing From Childhood Trauma

Francesca Gold

Table of Contents

INTRODUCTION 1

CHAPTER 1: THE IMPACT OF CHILDHOOD TRAUMA ON ADULT RELATIONSHIPS 7

MY OWN TOXIC FAMILY...8
A DEFINING MOMENT 9
PRAYING TO GET OUT OF THERE 11
MY WAY OUT 12

CHAPTER 2: DIFFERENCES AND SIMILARITIES BETWEEN NARCISSISTIC AND TOXIC FAMILIES 17

ARE TOXIC FAMILIES NARCISSISTIC?...................................18
The Nature of Toxic Families...18
The Nature of Narcissistic Families..................................19
The Overlap: How Toxic and Narcissistic Behaviors Intersect..20
Key Differences Between Toxic and Narcissistic Families 21
HOW TO PROTECT YOURSELF IN THESE ENVIRONMENTS...................22
WHAT IS NARCISSISTIC PERSONALITY DISORDER? 23
Common Traits and Symptoms of NPD................................24
Diagnostic Criteria for NPD (DSM-5)................................25
Challenges of Treating NPD 26
Protecting Your Well-Being...27

CHAPTER 3: WHY DO EMPATHS OFTEN END UP IN RELATIONSHIPS WITH NARCISSISTS 29

WHY DO EMPATHS OFTEN END UP IN RELATIONSHIPS WITH NARCISSISTS? 30
Why Do Empaths Attract Narcissists? 30
Why Do Narcissists Target Empaths?...............................32
RED FLAGS FOR EMPATHS 33

Protecting Yourself From a Narcissist 36

CHAPTER 4: CODEPENDENCY 39

Codependency 40
What Is Codependency? 40
Key Characteristics of Codependency 41
Types of Codependency 42
Causes and Risk Factors of Codependency 43
Signs You Might Be Codependent 45
Breaking Free From Codependency 46

CHAPTER 5: WHAT ARE ATTACHMENT STYLES? 51

What Are Attachment Styles? 52
Secure Attachment 52
Anxious-Preoccupied Attachment 53
Dismissive-Avoidant Attachment 54
Fearful-Avoidant Attachment 55
Additional Attachment Styles 56
Factors That Influence Attachment Styles 57
Impact of Attachment Styles on Relationships 59
Romantic Relationships 59
Friendships 60
Family Relationships 60
Work Relationships 61
Mental Health and Well-Being 61
Tips for Changing Attachment Style 61

CHAPTER 6: WHAT IS THE CONCEPT OF THE INNER CHILD? ...65

What Is the Concept of the Inner Child? 66
Aspects of the Inner Child 67
Origins of the Inner Child 68
Characteristics of the Inner Child 69
Impact of the Inner Child on Adulthood 70
Healing the Inner Child 71
Therapeutic Approaches for Healing 72
Self-Care Practices for Healing 73
Books to Guide Your Healing Journey 73

CHAPTER 7: HOW DO I HEAL MY INNER CHILD?................75

STEP 1: ACKNOWLEDGE AND ACCEPT 76
STEP 2: IDENTIFY AND EXPRESS EMOTIONS.........................77
STEP 3: REPARENTING...78
STEP 4: REFRAME NEGATIVE EXPERIENCES 79
STEP 5: INTEGRATE YOUR INNER CHILD 80
ADDITIONAL TECHNIQUES FOR HEALING 81
DO NOT HESITATE TO SEEK SUPPORT 82

CHAPTER 8: WHY DOES HEALING YOUR INNER CHILD RESULT IN ATTRACTING HEALTHIER RELATIONSHIPS? 85

HOW INNER HEALING REFLECTS ON THE OUTSIDE 86
HEALTHY RELATIONSHIP PATTERNS 88
NO LONGER ATTRACTING TOXIC PARTNERS 89
ATTRACTING NURTURING PARTNERS 90
SIGNS OF HEALING YOUR INNER CHILD 92
RELATIONSHIP BENEFITS OF HEALING YOUR INNER CHILD.........93

CHAPTER 9: FINDING LOVE THROUGHOUT YOUR HEALING JOURNEY 95

EMBRACING VULNERABILITY 96
NAVIGATING RELATIONSHIPS 97
MINDSET SHIFTS 98
SPIRITUAL CONNECTION 99

CHAPTER 10: LOVING YOURSELF WILL ALWAYS NEED TO BE YOUR HIGHEST PRIORITY 101

SELF-LOVE FOUNDATIONS...102
BENEFITS OF SELF-LOVE...103
PRACTICES FOR SELF-LOVE 105
OVERCOMING OBSTACLES...106
EMPOWERMENT THROUGH SELF-LOVE.............................107

CHAPTER 11: HOW TO RAISE YOUR CHILDREN SO THEY STAY CONNECTED WITH THEIR INNER CHILD AND LEARN TO NURTURE AND HEAL THEMSELVES FROM A YOUNG AGE ...111

BUILDING A FOUNDATION FOR EMOTIONAL SAFETY....................113

How to Create Emotional Safety 113
Teaching Self-Compassion From a Young Age 114
Ways to Teach Self-Compassion 115
The Power of Play and Creativity 116
Ways to Encourage Creativity and Play 117

FINAL THOUGHTS 119

REFERENCES 123

Introduction

Narcissism has more in common with self-hatred than with self-admiration. –Christopher Lasch

If you have opened this book, chances are you are feeling weary. Are you exhausted from being caught in a distressing loop, repeatedly finding yourself in relationships that leave you feeling depleted and shattered? Perhaps you have spent countless nights questioning why you are consistently drawn to individuals who harm you, leaving you feeling insignificant, unworthy, and invisible. You may even believe there is something inherently wrong with you— an inner force that keeps attracting narcissists and toxic personalities into your life.

But I want you to know that there is nothing wrong with you. The pain, heartache, and confusion you have felt are not your fault. You are not broken or beyond repair—you have simply been wounded, often in ways that began long before you were even aware of them. Because of those early wounds, you have come to believe you are not enough, that you must work to earn love, prove yourself worthy of care, and sacrifice your happiness to maintain peace in your relationships.

This book is for you—the one who feels lost, unseen, and misunderstood. It is for the person who has weathered the storm of narcissistic abuse and is now ready to step out of the chaos and into healing. Healing does not happen overnight, and it will not always be easy. But it is possible. And more importantly, you deserve it.

Narcissistic abuse is more than just a bad relationship. It is an experience that leaves you questioning your reality, your worth, and your ability to trust yourself. Narcissists are experts at making you doubt everything about yourself, twisting situations to make you feel like you are always in the wrong, no matter how hard you try. They manipulate your kindness, exploit your empathy, and leave you emotionally battered. It is isolating, and it can feel impossible to break free.

But here is the truth: You are not alone. Countless people, just like you, have found themselves trapped in these painful cycles. You may feel ashamed, thinking, "Why do I keep choosing people like this?" or "How did I let this happen again?" But shame does not belong to you; it belongs to the person who manipulated and hurt you. Recognizing this is the first step to reclaiming your power and finding your way back to yourself. We share a common journey of pain and healing.

In this book, we will explore not just the surface-level behaviors of narcissists, but also the deeper, often hidden wounds that keep drawing you into these relationships. Many of these wounds stem from your inner child—the part of you that was hurt long ago and still carries that pain today. By reconnecting with and healing that inner child, you will be able to break free from these patterns once and for all.

This book is more than just a guide; it is a lifeline. In the following pages, you will learn how to stop attracting toxic people into your life by healing the parts of yourself that have been conditioned to seek love in unhealthy ways.

Healing is a process, and this book will guide you every step of the way, offering advice and genuine understanding. Each chapter will take you deeper into the root causes of the pain you have experienced, showing you how to gently unravel it so you can finally live the life you deserve—one filled with love, joy, and peace.

You might wonder, "How do I know this book is right for me? How can this person possibly understand what I have been through?" I understand the hesitation. Trusting someone to guide you through such a vulnerable process is no small thing. So, let me share why I believe I can help you heal. I understand because I have been there. I have felt the pain, the confusion, and the longing for healing.

I did not grow up in a nurturing, loving family. My childhood was filled with chaos, fear, and emotional pain. I was the youngest of three children, but instead of being protected and cared for, I was often the target of my older brother's uncontrollable rage. My mother was terrified, my father was silent, and my childhood home felt more like a battleground than a safe space. I grew up feeling unsafe, unworthy, and alone.

As I got older, those early wounds did not just disappear; they followed me into adulthood, shaping every relationship I had. Like many of you, I found myself in a series of toxic relationships with people who made me feel small, powerless, and unlovable. I did not know how to stand up for myself. I did not know how to set boundaries or say "no" without feeling guilty. For years, I suffered in silence, battling depression and questioning whether I would ever find real love or happiness.

But something changed when I became a mother. For the first time, I experienced pure and unconditional love. It awakened something inside me—a fierce desire to heal, not just for myself but for my child. I realized that to give my daughter the love and safety she deserved, I had to first heal the little girl inside of me who had never felt safe, loved, or enough.

That was the beginning of my healing journey, and it was not easy. There were many lonely moments and nights when I questioned if I could do it. But with time, self-compassion, and a lot of inner work, I began to break free. I learned to love myself, set boundaries, and attract healthy, loving relationships. Now, after years of healing, I am not just surviving; I am thriving.

I know what it is like to feel trapped in a cycle of pain. I know how hard it is to believe that healing is possible after being hurt so many times. But I also know that healing is possible because I have lived it. And now, I want to share everything I have learned with you.

This book is an invitation to heal, grow, and reclaim the parts of yourself that may have been lost along the way. You are not too broken, damaged, or far gone to heal. You are capable of experiencing deep, transformative healing, and I am here to help guide you through it.

This book is not just a guide but a beacon of hope for your healing journey.

You are not alone. Let us take this journey together!

Chapter 1:

The Impact of Childhood Trauma on Adult Relationships

Narcissists are like parasitic bugs that leech onto you and essentially suck the life out of you, then when you are no longer useful, they discard you. It's called the narcissistic abuse cycle.
–Silvi Saxena

Growing up in a toxic family leaves wounds that can linger long after childhood. When the love, safety, and trust every child deserves are replaced by fear, neglect, or chaos, it shapes how you see the world and relate to others. Often, without realizing it, the survival patterns you developed as a child—staying quiet to avoid conflict, seeking approval to feel loved—carry into adulthood, keeping you trapped in painful, unhealthy relationships.

I know this because I lived it. The trauma I experienced in my early years became the foundation for many of my adult relationships, and for a long time, I did not understand why I kept ending up in the same toxic cycles. But there is hope. Healing the inner child can break these patterns and free you from the pain that has followed you for so long.

In this chapter, I will share moments from my childhood to illustrate how trauma can shape your relationships and, more importantly, how healing is possible. Keep reading—you are not alone on this journey.

My Own Toxic Family

I grew up in a beautiful village by the Mediterranean Sea, but despite the scenic surroundings, my childhood was anything but peaceful. I was the youngest of three children—my brother was ten years older, and my sister was just two years my senior. My parents ran a small hotel, and from a young age, my days were filled with helping around the property—making beds, assisting my mom in the kitchen, and serving tables with my dad. This routine became my life, every day, from morning until night, until I turned 26. School was my only real escape, and I clung to my studies as a safety net because books made sense to me in a way my home life never did.

While my parents worked hard to provide for us, it came at a huge cost: We did not have a healthy, happy family life. My oldest brother was at the center of much of our family's chaos. His outbursts were unpredictable, his temper terrifying. There was always yelling, arguing, and loud threats that made you shrink inside. Our hotel was not just a place of business; it was often a war zone, and I still remember the discomfort on the faces of guests who witnessed our family drama unfold.

My brother hated me, resenting me simply for existing. Being the youngest and receiving my father's affection only fueled his jealousy. He was cruel and angry, constantly looking for ways to intimidate us. He would lash out at my mom, sometimes even threatening her with violence, and never hesitated to hurl insults at my father. He blamed everyone but himself for his problems, refusing to seek help or take responsibility for anything. Despite their best intentions, my parents seemed helpless in the face of his rage. They had given him every opportunity—education, career support— but he let his insecurities and temper drive everyone away.

A Defining Moment

Looking back, it is hard to believe how much fear filled that house, how we tiptoed around his moods, always trying to avoid the next explosion. My brother's behavior shaped so much of who I became, and it took years to understand how deeply those early experiences impacted the relationships I formed later in life.

One defining moment from my childhood still haunts me. I was only eight years old, standing in the hotel kitchen, watching a scene no child should ever witness. My brother was holding a broom, threatening to hit my mom. She was crouched by the kitchen sink, terrified, trying to make herself as small as possible. My father was there, too, standing with his arms crossed, saying nothing, doing nothing. He just watched.

I remember feeling frozen with fear, filled with a deep sense of helplessness. My mom was crying, my brother was yelling like a madman, and my dad—he just stood there, doing nothing. No one was protecting her, and I could not bear it anymore. My heart was racing, but I knew I had to act. So, I screamed. I yelled at my brother, using words I had never dared say before, curse words I was not even sure I knew. I shouted for him to stop, to leave her alone. And for some reason, it worked. My brother stopped, shocked that I had dared to stand up to him. He put the broom down, and for the first time, I felt like I had saved my mom.

That moment changed me forever. It was not just about saving her; it was about realizing that I could not rely on anyone else to protect me or the people I loved. I made decisions that day—silent, subconscious ones— that shaped the rest of my life. I decided I would never allow myself to be vulnerable like that again. I looked at my father and saw weakness. I looked at my brother and saw danger. From that point forward, I believed that men were unreliable, unsafe, and incapable of protecting anyone.

That belief followed me into adulthood, into every relationship I had. The men I ended up with felt familiar—too familiar. They were toxic in their own ways, and I found myself feeling the same fear and helplessness I had as a child. Some relationships left me feeling emotionally unsafe, while others made me fear for my physical safety. Those early decisions, born from fear and a desperate need to protect myself, shaped so much of my life without me even realizing it.

Praying to Get Out of There

I never felt safe as a child. Every day brought a new wave of fear and uncertainty. I watched my mom cry more times than I can count, her spirit crushed under the weight of my brother's rage. My father was always silent, his strength drained by the constant abuse. And my sister? She seemed emotionally checked out, focused only on what she could take from the situation—always asking for money, always mean, especially to me.

From a very young age, I dreamed of escaping. I studied hard because school was the only place that felt stable. Books were logical and predictable in a way my home life never was. Math, science, English literature—these subjects brought me peace. School became my refuge, a place where I did not have to tiptoe around my family's fragile emotions. I buried myself in my studies, hoping that one day, they would be my ticket out of the chaos.

Every night, I would go to the bathroom, open the window, and pray. I would kneel, look up at the stars, and beg God to take me away from that life. I was not asking for anything extravagant—just a place where I could feel safe, where I could finally breathe without the constant weight of fear pressing down on my chest.

All I ever wanted was a real family, where love was not overshadowed by anger and fear.

When I reached high school, I thought I had found a way out. I met an Italian boy, and for a time, it felt like an escape. But after two years, he turned to drugs, and I knew I could not stay. That relationship ended, but it set a pattern that would follow me for years—choosing men who mirrored the chaos I had grown up with. I did not know how to set boundaries, did not know how to say "no" or demand respect. I kept finding myself in relationships where I felt small, powerless, and afraid.

The pain I carried from my childhood followed me into adulthood, fueling decades of depression. I did not know how to love myself, and without that foundation, I could not stand up for myself with the quiet confidence that comes from knowing your worth. And so, I cycled through one unhealthy relationship after another, never fully understanding why I kept ending up in the same painful situations.

My Way Out

Books were my sanctuary. They transported me to worlds where love, care, and compassion existed—far removed from the chaos of my home life. In those pages, I found comfort and safety. They gave me the strength to dream of a future where I could create a life that made sense and felt stable. I poured myself into my studies, knowing that education was my only way out.

I chose chemistry in college because it was precise and logical—everything my life was not. And I gave it my all. Graduating *cum laude* was not just an academic achievement for me; it was proof that I could create a future different from the one I had been handed. After that, I moved to England for my PhD and eventually to the United States to complete my postdoctoral work. I became a Research Assistant Professor, something I could never have imagined as a scared little girl kneeling by the bathroom window, praying for a way out.

I was the first in my entire extended family to graduate from college, the first to earn a PhD, and the first to publish in prestigious scientific journals. On paper, it looked like I had achieved everything. I had pulled myself out of that dark childhood and built a life I could be proud of. But despite all of my success, I was still deeply lonely. I had spent so many years chasing academic achievements that I had not realized I was carrying my childhood trauma with me. It showed up in other ways—in my relationships, in the quiet moments when loneliness crept in.

What I longed for, more than anything, was a family of my own—a partner who could love me the way I had never been loved. But that longing led me into relationships that mirrored the same pain I grew up with. I moved from one relationship to the next, each one filled with men who carried their own childhood wounds. Just like me, they did not know how to show love in a healthy way. Instead of the nurturing love I craved, I found myself tangled in toxic dynamics that felt all too familiar—relationships filled with emotional distance, manipulation, and pain. Without realizing it, I was still reliving the trauma of my childhood, repeating the patterns I had learned so young.

Then, at 40, I became a mother. For the first time in my life, I felt real, unconditional love. Holding my daughter in my arms changed everything. She brought a kind of love I had never experienced—a pure, innocent love that asked for nothing but to be cherished. But as beautiful as that moment was, it also came with heartbreak. Her father was a narcissist, and as much as I wanted to believe I could create a family with him, the relationship only brought more trauma. When I found myself pregnant and alone, I realized something had to change.

Being forced into that situation made me confront the deepest parts of myself. I could not keep running from my pain anymore. I had to heal, not just for me, but for my baby girl. I knew I could not give her the love and safety she deserved if I did not first heal the wounded child inside of me—the one who still felt unloved, scared, and unworthy.

Healing was not easy. There were lonely nights and moments when I questioned whether I could do this alone. But each time I looked at my daughter, I was reminded why it mattered so much. I had to break the cycle, not just for me but for her. I could not let my trauma define her life.

Little by little, I started to feel genuine love—not just for my daughter but for myself, too. I began to realize that I was worthy of love and did not have to settle for the familiar pain that had followed me for so long. In the healing process, I started to rebuild the most important relationship in my life—the one with myself.

That journey is still ongoing, but the difference now is that I am no longer running from my pain. I am facing it, healing it, and creating a new life for myself and my daughter—one filled with love, peace, and joy I never knew was possible.

In the next chapter, we will take a look at the differences and similarities between narcissistic and toxic families.

Chapter 2:

Differences and Similarities Between Narcissistic and Toxic Families

Love doesn't die a natural death; love has to be killed, either by neglect or narcissism. –Frank Salvato

Being in a relationship with narcissistic and toxic individuals can leave you feeling confused, broken, and questioning your reality. Narcissists may draw you in with charm, only to reveal their manipulative nature once you are deeply invested. But how do you know if someone is a narcissist? And what distinguishes a narcissistic relationship from a toxic one?

In this chapter, we will explore the traits that define narcissistic individuals and how they differ from those found in toxic but non-narcissistic families. While not all toxic families are led by narcissists, patterns of emotional abuse, control, and manipulation often overlap. We will break down the characteristics of narcissistic personality disorder (NPD) to help you recognize red flags in the people around you.

Understanding these traits is not about labeling others; it is about empowering yourself to recognize patterns and protect your emotional well-being. If you have ever felt something was off but could not quite identify it, this chapter will help you understand what is going on and why it is not your fault. Read on!

Are Toxic Families Narcissistic?

While toxic and narcissistic families often share the harm they cause, they are not the same. Both environments can feel suffocating and damaging, but not every toxic family centers around a narcissist, and not every narcissistic family is toxic in the same way. However, the overlapping patterns in both types of families leave lasting emotional scars.

The Nature of Toxic Families

Toxic families are marked by various destructive behaviors that can leave you feeling confused, unsafe, or emotionally depleted. These families may not have a single controlling figure, yet the environment remains harmful. Often, toxic family dynamics are shaped by emotional abuse, where love and care are conditional, leaving members constantly walking on eggshells.

Common traits of toxic families include:

- **Emotional abuse:** Frequent criticism, belittling, or verbal attacks that make you question your worth.

- **Manipulation:** Members twist situations or words to gain control, often making you feel responsible for their actions.

- **Gaslighting:** A subtle form of psychological manipulation that causes you to doubt your reality, leaving you confused and uncertain.

- **Control:** Tight control over decisions, feelings, or even your basic identity, often enforced through guilt or fear.

- **Lack of empathy:** An inability to understand or care about your feelings, leading to emotional neglect.

- **Favoritism:** Playing siblings or family members against each other, creating divisions and feelings of inadequacy.

- **Unpredictability:** Emotional highs and lows that leave you constantly uncertain about what is coming next.

The Nature of Narcissistic Families

When a narcissistic parent or caregiver leads a family, the dysfunction takes on a unique form. Narcissists are known for their inflated sense of self-importance, need for admiration, and lack of empathy. In narcissistic families, the desires and image of the narcissist come first, leaving others to manage the fallout.

Narcissistic families are often characterized by:

- **Emotional unavailability:** The narcissist focuses more on themselves than on the emotional needs of family members.

- **Self-centeredness:** The family revolves around the narcissist, leaving little room for others' feelings or experiences.

- **Manipulation:** The narcissist twists situations to maintain control, using either charm or cruelty to serve their interests.

- **Need for admiration:** Constant validation is sought, with the narcissist lashing out if they feel ignored.

- **Lack of empathy:** They cannot understand or care about the emotional pain they cause others.

The Overlap: How Toxic and Narcissistic Behaviors Intersect

In many cases, the lines between toxic and narcissistic families blur. Both environments are filled with emotional manipulation, lack of empathy, and control. In both, individual needs are sidelined to maintain a power dynamic, rooted either in dysfunction or narcissistic traits.

- **Emotional abuse and manipulation:** Both family types use emotional abuse as a control tool. Whether through cruelty or subtle manipulation, the result is often a sense of unworthiness, confusion, and emotional neglect.

- **Lack of empathy:** Members in both family types rarely prioritize others' feelings, leading to deep emotional wounds.

- **Control and dominance:** Control is central to both dynamics, enforced through fear, guilt, or manipulation to keep others emotionally subservient.

Key Differences Between Toxic and Narcissistic Families

One key difference is that toxic families are not always driven by a narcissistic personality disorder. In a toxic family, dysfunction may stem from poor communication skills, unresolved trauma, or emotional immaturity without a clear figure embodying narcissistic traits.

In a narcissistic family, however, one or more members (often a parent or sibling) display specific behaviors associated with narcissistic personality disorder (NPD). They see themselves as superior and expect admiration, often at the expense of others' well-being. Narcissistic families revolve around the narcissist's needs, with little regard for the impact on other members.

How to Protect Yourself in These Environments

If you are living in a toxic or narcissistic family, prioritizing your well-being is essential. Setting boundaries is one of the most powerful steps you can take. Boundaries protect your emotional space and allow you to say "no" to harmful behaviors. This can be challenging, especially if you are used to putting others' needs before your own, but it is a crucial step toward healing.

- **Practice self-care:** Dedicate moments each day to focus on yourself. This could be through journaling, mindfulness, or simply engaging in activities you enjoy. Self-care helps ground you and reinforces your self-worth.

- **Set boundaries:** Identify and assert limits with family members who are emotionally abusive or manipulative. This might include reducing contact or disengaging from conversations that drain you. Boundaries are about safeguarding your well-being, even if others resist or push back.

- **Seek support:** You do not have to navigate this alone. Reach out to trusted friends, support groups, or mental health professionals who can offer guidance and understanding as you manage the complexities of toxic or narcissistic family dynamics.

Remember, you deserve to feel safe and valued, even if your family environment did not teach you that. Healing is possible and starts with reclaiming your emotional health, one step at a time.

What Is Narcissistic Personality Disorder?

Narcissistic personality disorder (NPD) is more than just selfish or self-absorbed behavior; it is a serious mental health condition that profoundly impacts how a person interacts with others. People with NPD often have an exaggerated sense of self-importance, an intense need for admiration, and a troubling lack of empathy for those around them. They tend to see themselves as superior and may use manipulation and control to align others with their inflated sense of self.

The term "narcissism" comes from the ancient Greek myth of Narcissus, a young man who fell in love with his reflection. This serves as a fitting metaphor for NPD, where individuals are so focused on themselves that they struggle to connect meaningfully with others.

Common Traits and Symptoms of NPD

People with NPD often exhibit hallmark traits that can make relationships with them challenging. Their constant need for validation and lack of empathy create emotional distance, making it difficult for them to form meaningful connections and often leaving emotional damage in their wake.

Here are some common symptoms:

- **Grandiosity and self-importance:** They see themselves as special or superior.

- **Fixation on beauty, talent, or achievement:** They become obsessed with success or appearance, often at the expense of genuine connections.

- **Need for constant admiration:** Individuals with NPD crave attention and praise and may feel empty without it.

- **Sense of entitlement:** They believe they deserve special treatment and may react negatively if they do not receive it.

- **Lack of empathy:** They struggle to understand or care about others' feelings or needs.

- **Envy and resentment:** They often feel envious of others and believe others are envious of them.

- **Arrogant and haughty behavior:** They display a superior attitude and may be dismissive or condescending.

- **Difficulty handling criticism or failure:** Even minor criticism can trigger rage or lead to emotional withdrawal.

- **Manipulative and exploitative:** They use others to meet their own needs, often without guilt or remorse.

Diagnostic Criteria for NPD (DSM-5)

The *Diagnostic and Statistical Manual of Mental Disorders* (DSM-5) outlines specific criteria for diagnosing narcissistic personality disorder. To qualify, an individual must exhibit at least five of the following traits:

- A grandiose sense of self-importance (exaggerates achievements, expects to be recognized as superior without commensurate accomplishments).

- Preoccupation with fantasies of unlimited success, power, brilliance, beauty, or ideal love.

- A belief that they are "special" and unique and can only be understood by or associated with other special or high-status people.

- Need for excessive admiration.

- Sense of entitlement (unreasonable expectations of favorable treatment or compliance with their expectations).

- Interpersonal exploitation (taking advantage of others to achieve their own ends).

- Lack of empathy (unwillingness to recognize or identify with others' feelings and needs).

- Envy of others or belief that others are envious of them.

- Arrogant or haughty behaviors or attitudes.

These criteria provide mental health professionals with a guide to diagnosing NPD. However, it is essential to remember that only a trained expert can diagnose this disorder.

Challenges of Treating NPD

One major challenge in treating NPD is that individuals with the disorder rarely seek help voluntarily. They may not see their behavior as problematic, and even if they do, they are often unwilling to acknowledge their flaws. Therapy can be challenging because it requires self-reflection, which those with NPD may resist. However, with consistent treatment, including therapies like psychodynamic therapy or cognitive behavioral therapy (CBT), some individuals with NPD can learn to manage their symptoms better. These therapies focus on developing empathy, building healthier relationships, and challenging distorted self-perceptions.

If you are concerned that you or someone you care about might have NPD, reaching out to a mental health professional is crucial. Self-diagnosis can be misleading; only a trained expert can provide the clarity and support needed to navigate this complex condition.

Protecting Your Well-Being

If you are dealing with someone who has NPD, it is crucial to protect your own mental and emotional health. Prioritizing self-care and setting boundaries are essential steps to safeguard your well-being.

In understanding the characteristics of narcissists and the dynamics of toxic and narcissistic families, it becomes clear that recognizing these traits is key to protecting your emotional health. By identifying red flags and setting boundaries, you empower yourself to reclaim your sense of self and prioritize your mental well-being.

Have you ever wondered why empaths often end up in relationships with narcissists? The next chapter explains it all!

Chapter 3

Why Do Empaths Often End Up in Relationships With Narcissists

Sometimes it's not the people who change; it's the mask that falls off. –Haruki Murakami.

Have you ever wondered why, despite your best intentions and deeply caring nature, you keep finding yourself in relationships with people who drain you emotionally? As an empath, your ability to understand and feel others' emotions is a gift—but with narcissists, that very gift can become a trap. Narcissists are experts at charming their way into your life, only to later exploit your kindness, compassion, and vulnerability.

The unfortunate reality is that empaths and narcissists are often drawn to each other because their personalities, though seemingly opposite, fit together in a toxic way. Empaths want to heal and nurture, while narcissists crave attention and control. This combination can initially feel like an intense, whirlwind connection but often becomes suffocating and exhausting over time.

In this chapter, we will explore why empaths are particularly vulnerable to narcissists, how to recognize the red flags early on, and, most importantly, how to protect yourself from falling into the same patterns again.

Why Do Empaths Often End Up in Relationships With Narcissists?

Empaths and narcissists are often irresistibly drawn to each other, creating a connection that can feel electric at first—like the perfect match. However, over time, the relationship often turns toxic. Why does this happen? Despite being on opposite ends of the emotional spectrum, empaths and narcissists complement each other in a way that can be damaging. The empath gives endlessly, while the narcissist takes without limit. This dynamic, though harmful, can initially feel familiar or even comforting.

Why Do Empaths Attract Narcissists?

Empaths are naturally warm, caring, and emotionally available. They deeply understand others' feelings and often go out of their way to provide comfort and support. To a narcissist, this is magnetic. Narcissists are always seeking what is known as *narcissistic supply*—a constant flow of admiration, attention, and emotional fuel. An empath's emotional openness provides the perfect source for this, as they give selflessly, often without realizing how much they sacrifice.

Empaths' compassion also makes them more likely to tolerate a narcissist's toxic behaviors. Narcissists may reveal signs of emotional unavailability or manipulation early on, but empaths, with their boundless empathy, often believe they can help, understand, or even "heal" the narcissist. This desire for meaningful connection can keep the empath tethered to someone who promises emotional depth but never truly delivers.

Then, there is the matter of trust. Empaths tend to see the good in people and trust easily. Narcissists exploit this trust, using it to manipulate and control. In the relationship's early stages, narcissists often present themselves as caring, loving, and attentive—exactly what the empath is seeking. But as time passes, the facade falls away, and the narcissist's true, manipulative nature emerges. By the time the empath recognizes what is happening, they are often so emotionally invested that breaking free feels incredibly difficult.

Empaths are also naturally selfless, often prioritizing others' needs over their own, and narcissists take full advantage of this. The more the empath gives, the more the narcissist takes, leaving the empath drained and emotionally exhausted. Narcissists thrive on this dynamic, knowing the empath's desire to help will keep them locked in the cycle of giving.

Why Do Narcissists Target Empaths?

Narcissists are drawn to empaths because they provide exactly what the narcissist craves: emotional supply. Narcissists feed off attention, admiration, and validation, and empaths, with their compassionate nature, are often more than willing to provide it. The narcissist knows that the empath will continually give without expecting much in return, making it easy to manipulate and control the relationship.

Narcissists also thrive on control. An empath's sensitivity and willingness to put others first make them prime targets for manipulation. Narcissists use the empath's emotions against them, creating situations where the empath feels responsible for the narcissist's happiness or well-being. This control gives the narcissist a sense of power and reinforces their inflated self-image.

Another reason narcissists target empaths is the admiration they receive. Empaths are generous with praise and often see the potential in others, even when it is not immediately apparent. Narcissists feed off this admiration, using it to reinforce their sense of superiority. The empath's admiration becomes a mirror, reflecting the narcissist's idealized self-image.

Furthermore, narcissists use empaths as emotional regulators. When a narcissist feels insecure, angry, or emotionally unstable, they rely on the empath to soothe their emotions. The empath's calming presence stabilizes the narcissist's inner turmoil, but at a cost—draining the empath's emotional energy. The narcissist rarely offers this emotional support in return, leaving the empath depleted and overwhelmed.

In the end, the empath-narcissist relationship is one in which the empath gives endlessly, and the narcissist takes without limit. This cycle can only be broken when the empath recognizes the toxic dynamic and begins to prioritize their own well-being.

Red Flags for Empaths

As an empath, your ability to feel deeply and connect emotionally is one of your greatest strengths. However, it also makes you more vulnerable to manipulation by narcissists. Narcissists are skilled at creating an illusion of love and connection, especially in the early stages of a relationship, often sweeping you off your feet before you realize what is happening. But there are warning signs—red flags—that, if noticed early, can protect you from emotional pain and manipulation.

1. **Instant Intense Connection (Love Bombing)**

One of the most glaring red flags is when a relationship progresses too quickly. This is called *love bombing*. Narcissists may shower you with affection, attention, and even declarations of love right from the start. It feels like a whirlwind romance, but it is actually a tactic to gain your trust and emotional investment. If someone claims you are "the one" within weeks or places you on a pedestal before really getting to know you, something may be amiss. Real, healthy love takes time to develop.

2. Charm and Flattery

Narcissists can be incredibly charming, knowing exactly what to say to make you feel special. But it is important to ask yourself if the charm is genuine or merely a tactic to win you over. Excessive flattery is often used to distract you from their true intentions. Pay attention to whether their compliments feel authentic or seem exaggerated and manipulative.

3. Self-Centered Conversations

Narcissists love to talk—about themselves. They dominate discussions, often steering them back to their own achievements, feelings, or needs. While they may show interest in you initially, it is usually superficial. Over time, you will notice the relationship revolves around them, and they rarely show genuine curiosity about your thoughts or emotions.

4. Emotional Unavailability

Though narcissists may seem emotionally engaged early on, their true emotional unavailability eventually becomes clear. They struggle with deeper connections and often shut down when asked to be vulnerable or discuss feelings. They will dodge emotional conversations or change the subject, leaving you feeling isolated in your own emotions.

5. Gaslighting, Manipulation, or Exploitation

Gaslighting is a form of emotional manipulation where the narcissist makes you question your reality. They may deny things they have said or done, or accuse you of being overly sensitive or irrational. This tactic is meant to confuse you and make you doubt your perceptions, giving them more control. Over time, this emotional manipulation can erode your self-esteem, making it harder to trust yourself.

6. Disregard for Boundaries

Narcissists often push boundaries, ignoring your requests for space or privacy. They may belittle your needs or make you feel guilty for setting limits. Healthy relationships require mutual respect, and if someone consistently crosses your boundaries or pressures you to compromise your values, it is a significant warning sign.

7. Grandiose Claims or Expectations

Narcissists often make grandiose claims about themselves, their ambitions, or their future plans. They will promise things that seem almost too good to be true—and often, they are. These exaggerated promises are meant to keep you hooked, always waiting for their fulfillment. In reality, however, they rarely follow through.

Protecting Yourself From a Narcissist

Once you have recognized these red flags, the next step is to protect yourself from getting entangled in a toxic relationship. As an empath, it is easy to put others' needs ahead of your own, but protecting your emotional health is essential.

1. Recognize Red Flags

Being aware of red flags is not just about looking back on past experiences; it is about catching them early on. Trust your gut feelings. If something feels off, do not ignore it. Empaths often have a strong intuition, but it is easy to dismiss those feelings when emotions are involved. Trust yourself, and do not hesitate to step back and evaluate the relationship.

2. Set Clear Boundaries

Learn to set boundaries early in any relationship. Boundaries are not about controlling others; they are about safeguarding your well-being. Be firm about what you will and will not tolerate—whether it is how you expect to be treated or how much emotional energy you are willing to invest. If someone repeatedly disregards your boundaries, it is a clear sign to distance yourself.

3. Prioritize Self-Care and Self-Awareness

Taking care of yourself is vital for maintaining healthy relationships. Self-care can mean anything from relaxing and recharging to seeking therapy or journaling. The more you invest in yourself, the more likely you will recognize when someone is not treating you right. Building emotional self-awareness will help you avoid losing yourself in a relationship.

4. **Do Not Tolerate Emotional Abuse**

No matter how much empathy you have, emotional abuse is never acceptable. Whether it is gaslighting, manipulation, or any other toxic behavior, you deserve better. Do not excuse or rationalize someone's actions just because you feel compassion for them. Your emotional health matters, and staying in an abusive relationship will only cause more harm.

5. **Seek Support From Trusted Friends, Family, or a Therapist**

It can be hard to see the full picture when you are in the middle of a relationship. That is why having a support system is so important. Talk to friends or family members you trust and who have your best interests at heart. If needed, seek help from a therapist who can provide guidance and help you navigate the complexities of dealing with a narcissist.

6. **Practice Self-Compassion and Self-Forgiveness**

As an empath, you might blame yourself for not recognizing the signs earlier or for staying in a toxic relationship too long. But remember, you acted out of love and care. Be kind to yourself. Healing is a journey, and it is okay to forgive yourself for past choices. What matters now is prioritizing your well-being and making choices that support your emotional health moving forward.

As an empath, you deserve relationships that nurture and support you. Trust your instincts, recognize when someone is not treating you with love and respect, and take steps to protect your emotional well-being. By setting boundaries and practicing self-care, you can break free from toxic patterns and find relationships that allow you to flourish. Empaths often give so much to others—now it is time to give that love and care back to yourself.

The next chapter will explore codependence, its various forms, and the risks it brings. You will discover how it develops and learn practical steps to build healthier, independent relationships.

Chapter 4:

Codependency

Worrying, obsessing, and controlling are illusions. They are tricks we play on ourselves. –Melody Beattie

Have you ever felt like you have lost yourself in your relationships—constantly putting your partner's needs above your own, worrying about their happiness more than your own, and feeling unable to say "no" for fear of abandonment? This pattern, known as codependency, is more common than you might think, especially if you have experienced toxic relationships or challenging family dynamics growing up. It can feel like you are stuck, unable to detach from the relationship, even when it is hurting you.

In this chapter, we will explore what codependency really is—why it happens, the signs to watch for, and how to break free. You will learn how childhood trauma and past relationship experiences can shape your attachment style and influence the relationships you choose. Most importantly, we will discuss how to reclaim your sense of self, set healthy boundaries, and build more balanced, fulfilling connections. Keep reading—it is time to break the cycle.

Codependency

Our attachment styles, shaped largely by early life experiences, play a significant role in how we form relationships as adults. For many, these attachment patterns can lead to codependency—a cycle of unhealthy emotional reliance on others that leaves us feeling trapped, drained, and stuck in relationships that do not serve our well-being.

What Is Codependency?

Codependency occurs when one person becomes excessively dependent on another for emotional validation, identity, or self-worth. In these relationships, the codependent person often puts their partner's needs above their own, sometimes without even realizing it. For example, you might constantly worry about how your partner feels, adjusting your behavior to keep them happy—even at the expense of your own comfort. This need for connection and approval can become overwhelming, leaving little room for your own emotional needs.

Codependency is not limited to romantic relationships. It can also occur between friends, family members, or colleagues. The common thread is an imbalance, where one person feels responsible for another's happiness and struggles to prioritize their own well-being.

Key Characteristics of Codependency

Here are some key traits of a codependent relationship:

- **Excessive emotional reliance on the other person:** You rely heavily on your partner to feel emotionally secure, making their feelings and moods your constant focus.

- **Enabling or supporting harmful behaviors:** You might ignore or even support your partner's destructive habits because you fear conflict or rejection.

- **Lack of boundaries and self-care:** You struggle to set personal boundaries and neglect your own needs.

- **Fear of abandonment or rejection:** The thought of being left alone feels unbearable, causing you to cling to relationships—even unhealthy ones.

- **Need for control or fixation on the other person:** You may feel the need to manage your partner's life, decisions, or emotions to maintain stability in the relationship.

- **Difficulty expressing your own needs and desires:** You find it hard to ask for what you need or want, fearing it will cause conflict.

- **Tendency to please others and sacrifice your well-being:** You constantly put others' needs ahead of your own, even when it exhausts or hurts you.

- **Inability to detach or set healthy limits:** Letting go feels impossible, even when the relationship is harmful.

- **Obsessive thinking about the other person:** You constantly worry about how they feel or what they think, often at the expense of your own peace of mind.

- **Feeling trapped or stuck in the relationship:** You may know the relationship is unhealthy, but feel powerless to leave.

Types of Codependency

Below are the most common types of codependency and the key features of each:

1. Active Codependency

Active codependency occurs when you take on the role of caregiver or fixer in the relationship. You may feel responsible for solving your partner's problems—whether they are emotional, financial, or related to addiction. This often comes at the cost of your own needs and well-being. For example, you might sacrifice your time, energy, or resources to help your partner, even when it drains you.

2. **Passive Codependency**

Passive codependency is subtler but equally damaging. In this case, you enable harmful behaviors by remaining silent or avoiding confrontation. You may allow your partner's negative actions to slide in order to prevent conflict, but in doing so, you sacrifice your emotional safety. It is a form of "going along to get along," but at the expense of your own mental health.

3. **Anxious Codependency**

Anxious codependency is driven by fear. You might try to control your partner's actions or emotions because you are terrified of abandonment. This often leads to clingy or overbearing behavior as you attempt to ensure your partner will not leave. It is exhausting for both people involved and can create even more tension in the relationship.

4. **Avoidant Codependency**

On the flip side, avoidant codependency happens when someone uses emotional distance to cope with the fear of intimacy. You might avoid deep connections or push your partner away because you fear getting too close and getting hurt. This fear of vulnerability prevents you from experiencing true emotional intimacy, even though, deep down, that is what you crave.

Causes and Risk Factors of Codependency

Codependency often stems from early life experiences and relationships that condition us to seek validation from others while neglecting our own needs. Here are some major causes:

- **Childhood trauma or neglect:** If you grew up in an environment where your emotional needs were not met, you may have learned to prioritize others in order to feel a sense of worth.

- **Family dynamics:** Growing up in families marked by addiction, abuse, or emotional neglect can teach you that love is conditional and that you must sacrifice yourself to maintain relationships.

- **Low self-esteem:** When you do not believe that you are enough, it is easy to seek validation from others—even when it comes at the expense of your own well-being.

- **Fear of abandonment:** Past experiences of being left or rejected can lead to an overwhelming fear of abandonment, making you cling to relationships, even unhealthy ones.

- **Past relationship trauma:** If you have been in relationships where your boundaries were disrespected or you were made to feel responsible for someone else's happiness, codependency can become a survival mechanism.

Signs You Might Be Codependent

Recognizing the signs of codependency is essential for breaking the cycle and regaining control of your emotional well-being. If any of these resonate with you, it might be time to reassess your relationships and how you engage in them.

- **Constant worry about your partner's emotions or actions:** If you find yourself frequently anxious about how your partner is feeling or what they are doing, it may be a sign of codependency. You might be hyper-aware of their moods, adjusting your behavior to prevent conflict or maintain peace. This constant worry often leads to emotional exhaustion and a lack of focus on your own needs.

- **Sacrificing your own needs and desires for your partner:** In a codependent relationship, it is common to prioritize your partner's needs over your own—even when it negatively impacts you. You might give up things that bring you joy or comfort, believing it will make your partner happier. Over time, this self-sacrifice leads to resentment, burnout, and a diminished sense of self.

- **Feeling responsible for your partner's happiness:** One of the hallmarks of codependency is feeling responsible for how your partner feels. If they are upset or stressed, you believe you must fix it—even if their emotional state has nothing to do with you.

This belief creates an unhealthy dynamic, where you take on their burdens and neglect your own emotional well-being.

- **Difficulty saying "no" or setting boundaries:** Codependent individuals often struggle with asserting themselves, especially when it comes to setting boundaries. You might fear that saying "no" will lead to conflict, disappointment, or abandonment. As a result, you end up agreeing to things you are uncomfortable with, which only further entrenches the imbalance in the relationship.

- **Feeling trapped or stuck in the relationship:** Even if you recognize that the relationship is not healthy, you might feel unable to leave. This feeling of being trapped is a common sign of codependency. You may fear being alone or believe you will not find another relationship, so you stay—even when it is clear that staying is harming you.

Breaking Free From Codependency

Breaking free from codependency is not easy, but with the right tools and mindset, it is possible. The following steps can help you regain independence, build healthier relationships, and improve your emotional well-being.

1. Self-Reflection and Awareness

The first step toward breaking free from codependency is recognizing the patterns. Take time to reflect on how your relationships have played out. Are there recurring themes of emotional dependence or self-sacrifice? Journaling or talking to a trusted friend can help you clarify your behaviors and understand why they developed in the first place.

2. Seeking Professional Help

Therapy, especially with someone who understands codependency, can be a powerful tool in your healing journey. A therapist can help you explore the root causes of your codependency, provide strategies for setting boundaries, and guide you toward healthier ways of relating. Counseling offers a safe space to process your emotions and build self-awareness.

3. Setting Healthy Boundaries

Learning to set boundaries is one of the most important steps in overcoming codependency. Start by identifying your own needs and limits. Practice saying "no" when something does not feel right, and communicate your boundaries clearly and respectfully. Setting boundaries does not make you selfish; it is a form of self-care that protects your emotional health.

4. Practicing Self-Care and Self-Compassion

Codependency often stems from neglecting your own needs. Prioritize self-care by engaging in activities that make you feel good, such as taking walks, reading, or simply spending time alone. Equally important is practicing self-compassion—be kind to yourself as you navigate this process. Healing takes time, and it is okay to stumble along the way.

5. Building Self-Esteem and Confidence

Many people struggling with codependency have low self-esteem, often because their sense of worth is tied to the approval or validation of others. Focus on building confidence by celebrating your strengths and achievements, no matter how small. Surround yourself with supportive people, and remind yourself that you are worthy of love and respect, independent of anyone else.

6. Developing Emotional Intelligence

Emotional intelligence—the ability to understand and manage your emotions—is key to breaking free from codependency. Learn to recognize when you feel overwhelmed, anxious, or overly invested in someone else's emotions. Practicing mindfulness and self-awareness can help you detach from the emotional highs and lows of others, allowing you to stay grounded in your own feelings.

7. Learning Healthy Communication Skills

Open and honest communication is essential in any relationship, especially when breaking free from codependent tendencies. Practice expressing your needs and feelings without fear of judgment or rejection. Healthy communication fosters mutual respect and understanding, creating space for both partners to grow individually and together.

Codependency can feel overwhelming, but recognizing the patterns is the first step toward change. Healing means prioritizing your well-being, setting boundaries, and regaining your sense of self. Remember, you are not responsible for someone else's happiness—your emotional health matters, too.

Breaking free takes time and self-compassion, but you can create healthier, more balanced relationships with patience, support, and a commitment to self-care. You deserve love and respect, both from others and yourself.

In the next chapter, we will explore the different attachment styles and their impact on relationships.

Chapter 5:

What Are Attachment Styles?

Attachment style is no different from any other human characteristic. Although we all have a basic need to form close bonds, the way we create them varies.
–Amir Levine & Rachel Heller

Have you ever wondered why some people seem so secure and comfortable in their relationships, while others struggle with a constant fear of abandonment or avoid intimacy altogether? The way we form and maintain relationships is often shaped by something deeper than conscious choice—our attachment style. This pattern begins in childhood and profoundly influences how we connect with others.

Attachment styles explain why we react the way we do in relationships. Understanding your attachment style can unlock many answers, whether you feel anxious when your partner is distant or prefer to keep people at arm's length. These patterns are not set in stone—they reflect our early experiences with caregivers, but they can shift with self-awareness and healing.

In this chapter, we will discuss the main attachment styles and how they impact your relationships.

What Are Attachment Styles?

Attachment styles are emotional patterns we develop in early childhood based on our relationships with caregivers. These styles strongly influence how we connect with others as adults, shaping our romantic relationships, friendships, and family bonds. Depending on the emotional availability and consistency of our caregivers, we may develop secure, anxious, avoidant, or fearful attachment styles, which affect how we respond to love, conflict, and intimacy.

Secure Attachment

People with a secure attachment style are comfortable with both intimacy and independence. They trust easily, communicate openly, and are unafraid of vulnerability in relationships. Because they experienced consistent care and responsiveness from their caregivers, they have learned that relationships can be safe and dependable.

For example, imagine someone who grew up with supportive parents who comforted her when she was upset but also encouraged her independence. As an adult, she is in a healthy relationship where she can openly express her feelings and give her partner space when needed. She knows that love and personal boundaries can coexist peacefully.

Key Traits of Secure Attachment:

- Comfortable with closeness and independence.

- Trusts easily and communicates openly.

- Manages conflict effectively.

- Emotionally resilient and adaptable.

- Regulates emotions in healthy ways.

Anxious-Preoccupied Attachment

People with an anxious-preoccupied attachment style tend to be sensitive and emotional in relationships. They often fear abandonment and worry that their partner may not feel as strongly as they do. This usually stems from childhood experiences with inconsistent caregivers—sometimes emotionally available, other times distant. As a result, they grow up uncertain of their worth and overly dependent on reassurance from others.

Consider someone who frequently checks on her partner and feels anxious without an immediate response. If her partner seems distant, she might assume something is wrong or fear abandonment, leading her to cling even more. Her fear of rejection often causes her to become overly attached and emotionally dependent.

Key Traits of Anxious-Preoccupied Attachment:

- Fear of rejection and abandonment.

- Overly dependent on a partner for emotional security.

- Prone to intense emotional reactions.

- Difficulty trusting their partner's love or intentions.

- Experiences high levels of anxiety in relationships.

Dismissive-Avoidant Attachment

Dismissive-avoidant individuals value independence to the extent that they avoid emotional closeness. As children, they may have had emotionally distant caregivers, which taught them not to rely on others. This leads them to prioritize self-reliance and avoid intimacy to protect themselves from potential hurt.

Imagine someone who values her independence so much that she avoids deep emotional connections. She feels uncomfortable when her partner tries to get close and prefers to keep her emotions to herself. This person may appear detached because she has learned to suppress her needs, fearing that relying on others leads to disappointment.

Key Traits of Dismissive-Avoidant Attachment:

- Prefers emotional distance and avoids intimacy.

- Values self-reliance over relationships.

- Suppresses emotions and avoids vulnerability.

- Struggles with emotional expression and connection.

- May seem distant or aloof in relationships.

Fearful-Avoidant Attachment

People with a fearful-avoidant attachment style experience a complex mix of wanting closeness but also fearing it. They may desire emotional connection yet push others away due to a fear of rejection or abandonment. This attachment style often develops in individuals who have experienced trauma, neglect, or inconsistent caregiving in childhood. They have learned that relationships can be both comforting and risky, leading to emotional dysregulation and internal conflict.

Imagine someone who deeply craves a loving relationship but feels overwhelming fear when things get too close. Though they may feel safe one moment, they become anxious the next, often withdrawing or sabotaging the relationship to avoid potential hurt. Their lack of trust and emotional instability make relationships difficult and painful.

Key Traits of Fearful-Avoidant Attachment:

- Fearful of both intimacy and abandonment.

- Difficulty trusting others and maintaining stable relationships.

- Experiences emotional highs and lows.

- Struggles with emotional regulation, especially in conflict.

- May have a history of trauma, abuse, or neglect.

Additional Attachment Styles

While the four main attachment styles (secure, anxious-preoccupied, dismissive-avoidant, and fearful-avoidant) are the most commonly discussed, other attachment forms can develop, especially in cases of severe trauma or inconsistent caregiving.

Disorganized-Disoriented Attachment

Disorganized-disoriented attachment is often trauma-related and marked by inconsistent or contradictory behaviors in relationships. Individuals with this attachment style may exhibit both anxious and avoidant tendencies, leading to confusion about their own feelings and actions. They may long for closeness but act in ways that unintentionally push others away, resulting in unpredictable relationship patterns. This attachment style often arises from situations where caregivers were a source of both comfort and fear, creating internal conflict about trust and safety in relationships.

Ambivalent Attachment

Ambivalent attachment combines elements of both anxious and avoidant traits. People with ambivalent attachment often experience conflicting emotions about their relationships—they desire closeness yet feel uncertain or hesitant about it. This internal conflict can lead to a push-and-pull dynamic in their relationships, where they feel torn between a fear of intimacy and a need for connection. As a result, they may seem inconsistent or unpredictable in how they relate to others, struggling to balance their conflicting desires.

Factors That Influence Attachment Styles

Attachment styles are shaped by various life experiences, especially in early childhood. These factors significantly impact how we form and maintain relationships throughout our lives.

1. **Early Childhood Experiences With Caregivers**

Our earliest relationships—those with our primary caregivers—lay the foundation for how we connect with others. When caregivers are emotionally available, nurturing, and responsive, we learn that relationships can be safe and reliable. In contrast, inconsistent or neglectful caregiving may lead us to question if others can be trusted. For example, a child who is comforted when distressed learns that their emotions are valued, whereas a child who is ignored may grow up feeling that their feelings do not matter.

2. Parenting Styles (Responsive, Sensitive, Consistent)

Parents who provide consistent, sensitive, and responsive care play a crucial role in fostering secure attachment. When a parent is attuned to a child's needs—offering comfort while encouraging independence—the child feels emotionally secure. Conversely, inconsistent parenting, where a parent's attentiveness fluctuates, can lead a child to feel anxious or avoidant, uncertain if their needs will be met. For instance, a child with an intermittently responsive parent may become clingy or fearful of abandonment.

3. Trauma or Neglect

Childhood trauma or neglect can significantly hinder the development of a healthy attachment style. A child who experiences abuse, neglect, or inconsistent caregiving may internalize feelings of fear, shame, or mistrust. Such experiences often result in attachment styles where relationships are associated with pain or loss. Trauma frequently leads to avoidant or fearful-avoidant attachment, as individuals may both crave connection and simultaneously fear the vulnerability it entails.

4. Attachment Experiences in Significant Relationships

Attachment styles can evolve in adulthood based on experiences in significant relationships. For example, a previously secure individual may develop attachment issues after a toxic or traumatic relationship, while someone with an insecure attachment can become more secure through a healthy, supportive partnership. How safe, valued, and supported we feel in these relationships plays a key role. A patient and understanding partner can help reduce an anxious person's fears, whereas a toxic relationship may intensify insecurities.

Impact of Attachment Styles on Relationships

Your attachment style significantly influences various types of relationships, affecting how you connect with others and respond to emotional needs.

Romantic Relationships

Attachment styles are most noticeable in romantic relationships. For example, a person with a secure attachment typically feels at ease with both intimacy and independence, able to trust their partner and communicate openly. In contrast, someone with an anxious attachment style may frequently seek reassurance, fearing abandonment and feeling insecure if their partner seems emotionally distant. Avoidant individuals, however, often struggle with closeness, preferring emotional distance, which can be challenging for a partner who seeks a deeper connection.

Friendships

Attachment styles also play a role in friendships. A securely attached person is likely to have stable, balanced friendships, with mutual support and reliability. In contrast, those with an anxious attachment may worry about being excluded or unloved by their friends, sometimes leading to overcompensation, like trying too hard to please. Avoidant individuals, on the other hand, might shy away from deep connections, opting instead for more casual, surface-level interactions.

Family Relationships

Attachment styles can either strengthen or complicate family dynamics. Secure individuals tend to maintain healthy boundaries while staying emotionally connected to family. Anxious attachment may lead to enmeshment, where individuals feel overly responsible for family members' emotions. Avoidant attachment can create emotional distance, with individuals shutting down or withdrawing when family members seek support.

Work Relationships

Attachment styles influence professional interactions and team dynamics as well. Securely attached individuals generally excel at balanced collaboration and communication. Those with an anxious attachment style may seek constant validation from coworkers or supervisors, fearing they are not performing adequately. Avoidant individuals often prefer working independently, avoiding emotional ties with colleagues, and sometimes resisting teamwork.

Mental Health and Well-Being

Attachment styles also impact mental health. Securely attached individuals tend to have higher self-esteem, emotional resilience, and balanced relationships. Conversely, insecure attachment styles can contribute to mental health challenges such as anxiety, depression, and self-doubt. Anxiously attached individuals may struggle with constant worry and feelings of inadequacy, while avoidant individuals might experience loneliness and emotional suppression, both of which can undermine overall well-being over time.

Tips for Changing Attachment Style

The good news is that attachment styles are not fixed. With self-awareness, effort, and the right support, you can work toward developing a more secure attachment style.

1. Self-Reflection and Awareness

The first step in changing your attachment style is understanding its origins. Reflect on how your childhood experiences have shaped your current relationship patterns. Recognizing your triggers—such as a fear of abandonment or discomfort with closeness—can help you start to shift your responses. Journaling or talking with a trusted friend can provide insight into the emotional patterns that no longer serve you.

2. Therapy (Individual, Couples, or Attachment-Focused)

Therapy is one of the most effective ways to address attachment issues. Individual therapy can help you explore the root causes of your attachment style and develop healthier emotional responses. Couples therapy improves relationship dynamics by helping both partners understand and work with their attachment styles. Therapies that focus specifically on attachment, such as Emotionally Focused Therapy (EFT), are especially effective for addressing insecure attachment patterns.

3. Healthy Relationships and Social Support

Surrounding yourself with supportive, healthy relationships is crucial for developing a secure attachment style. Positive, stable relationships with friends, family, or a romantic partner can provide the emotional security needed to heal from past experiences. When you feel safe, valued, and loved, it becomes easier to trust others and move beyond anxious or avoidant behaviors.

4. Mindfulness and Emotional Regulation Practices

Mindfulness can help you become more aware of your emotional triggers and reactions, teaching you to recognize when you are slipping into old attachment patterns—like seeking constant reassurance or emotionally withdrawing. Emotional regulation techniques, such as deep breathing or meditation, can help calm anxious feelings, giving you space to respond thoughtfully rather than react impulsively.

5. Self-Care and Personal Growth

Changing your attachment style also involves building a strong relationship with yourself. Focus on self-care by nurturing your mental and physical well-being. Activities that build your confidence, such as pursuing hobbies, setting personal goals, or practicing self-compassion, can enhance your sense of self-worth. As you grow and take care of yourself, you will be better equipped to form healthier, more balanced relationships with others.

By recognizing your attachment style and making intentional changes, you can break free from old patterns and build deeper connections rooted in trust, security, and emotional balance. Curious about your attachment style? Take a quick quiz through this link:

https://www.attachmentproject.com/attachment-style-quiz/

In the next chapter, we will dive into the concept of the "inner child"—an aspect of ourselves that can deeply influence our adult relationships. Understanding and nurturing this part of yourself can be a transformative step in creating more fulfilling, secure connections. Let us explore how reconnecting with your inner child can enhance your emotional well-being and relational health.

Chapter 6

What Is the Concept of the Inner Child?

The most sophisticated people I've ever known had one thing in common: they were all in touch with their inner children.
—Jim Henson

Have you ever noticed moments when you react to situations in a way that feels out of proportion, or when deep emotions surface unexpectedly? That is often your inner child at play—the part of you that holds onto childhood experiences, memories, and emotions. The inner child is not just a metaphor; it is a powerful psychological concept that represents the vulnerability, innocence, and emotional sensitivity we carry from our younger years into adulthood. Whether it is feelings of joy and playfulness or unresolved hurt and unmet needs, your inner child shapes how you respond to life's challenges and relationships.

For many of us, this part of our psyche may carry wounds, especially if we have experienced trauma, neglect, or emotional pain during our formative years. Those early experiences can leave us feeling emotionally reactive, fearful of abandonment, or struggling with self-worth. But here is the good news: Connecting with and healing your inner child can transform how you experience life today.

In this chapter, we will explore what the inner child is, how it impacts your adult self, and, most importantly, how to begin the journey of healing and reparenting the parts of you that still carry those childhood wounds.

What Is the Concept of the Inner Child?

The inner child is a psychological concept referring to the part of your subconscious that still holds onto childhood thoughts, feelings, and experiences. While you have grown into an adult, your inner child carries both positive and negative memories that continue to shape how you interact with the world today. Think of it as the part of you that remains vulnerable, curious, and sensitive but also holds unresolved pain or unmet needs.

For example, have you ever reacted emotionally to something minor, like feeling abandoned when someone does not text back? This might be your inner child responding, triggered by old feelings of rejection or loneliness. Understanding your inner child can give you insight into why certain emotions arise or why you behave in ways that seem irrational in adulthood.

Aspects of the Inner Child

Your inner child encompasses various qualities, many of which are rooted in your childhood self. Here are some core aspects of the inner child:

- **Vulnerability and innocence:** When life becomes overwhelming, this part of you feels small and exposed. It is where your most tender emotions reside—those that seek safety and care.

- **Emotional sensitivity:** Your inner child may overreact to criticism, neglect, or rejection, often surfacing in moments of hurt.

- **Creativity and playfulness:** The joy of being imaginative, spontaneous, and free is a hallmark of your inner child, reminding you that life is not only about responsibility.

- **Curiosity and wonder:** Remember the amazement you had as a child when everything felt new and exciting? That sense of wonder still exists within your inner child.

- **Unmet needs and unresolved emotions:** If you grew up in an environment where emotional needs were not met, these unfulfilled desires stay with you and may manifest in adult behaviors.

- **Memories and experiences (both positive and traumatic):** Your inner child holds onto memories of joy and trauma. These experiences—whether playing outside or experiencing neglect—remain a deep part of who you are.

Origins of the Inner Child

Early childhood experiences shape the development of your inner child. During this period, your psyche absorbs the emotions and dynamics around you.

- **Childhood experiences:** Trauma, neglect, or even the positive experiences of love and nurturing shape how your inner child feels about safety and connection.

- **Developmental stages:** Events like attachment, separation from caregivers, and key developmental milestones influence how your inner child internalizes the world.

- **Family dynamics and relationships:** How your family communicates, handles emotions, and shows affection impacts the behavior of your inner child. A nurturing environment fosters security, while a dysfunctional one can lead to fear and emotional isolation. For instance, if your parents were emotionally distant or you experienced neglect, your inner child might grow up feeling unworthy of love or afraid of abandonment, carrying these wounds into adult relationships.

Characteristics of the Inner Child

The inner child has certain traits that often manifest in adult life, especially when emotions are triggered.

- **Emotional reactivity:** Your inner child may respond intensely to situations that evoke old, unresolved feelings, sometimes leading to irrational or heightened emotional responses.

- **Impulsivity:** This part of you may act without thinking, much like a child would. It can show up in impulsive decisions or reactions driven by raw emotions.

- **Self-centeredness:** Children naturally view the world through their own needs and emotions. Your inner child might cause you to behave in more self-focused or dependent ways.

- **Dependence on others:** Your inner child may still seek approval, validation, or emotional security from external sources, much like a child depends on caregivers.

- **Fear of abandonment:** This is one of the strongest characteristics of a wounded inner child. A deep-rooted fear of being left or feeling unimportant often leads to insecurity in adult relationships.

Impact of the Inner Child on Adulthood

The inner child can significantly affect how you handle emotions, relationships, and overall well-being. Here are some ways it influences adulthood:

- **Emotional regulation difficulties:** A wounded inner child may struggle with managing emotions healthily, swinging between extreme responses, or shutting down entirely.

- **Relationship patterns:** Codependency, trust issues, or fear of intimacy often stem from unresolved childhood emotions carried by the inner child. For example, someone who grew up in an unstable home might feel anxious or clingy in relationships as an adult.

- **Self-esteem and confidence issues:** A wounded inner child often feels "not good enough," which may manifest as low self-esteem or a lack of confidence in adulthood.

- **Addictions or compulsive behaviors:** Some people cope with unresolved inner child pain through addictions or unhealthy behaviors like overeating, drinking, or compulsive shopping.

- **Physical and mental health problems:** Repressed childhood emotions can contribute to stress-related illnesses, anxiety, and depression.

Healing the Inner Child

Healing your inner child is a compassionate process of acknowledging your past and nurturing the parts of yourself that still feel wounded.

- **Acknowledge and accept your inner child:** The first step is recognizing that your inner child exists and their feelings are valid. You might begin this process through reflection or speaking with a therapist.

- **Identify unresolved emotions and needs:** Consider which unmet needs or feelings from childhood still affect you. Have you ignored emotions like fear, anger, or sadness?

- **Reparenting:** This is the act of becoming your own caregiver. Provide yourself with the love, validation, and care you may not have received as a child.

- **Reframe negative self-talk:** Your inner child may have internalized beliefs like "I am not good enough" or "I do not deserve love." Learn to replace these with affirmations of self-worth.

- **Integrate childhood experiences into adult awareness:** Allow your adult self to acknowledge your childhood experiences without letting them dictate your life now.

- **Seek professional help:** Therapists, particularly those specializing in trauma or inner child work, can guide you through the healing process.

Therapeutic Approaches for Healing

Various therapeutic approaches can help you heal your inner child and address unresolved trauma.

- **Inner child therapy:** Focuses on connecting with and nurturing the inner child to resolve childhood wounds.

- **Gestalt therapy:** Emphasizes living fully in the present moment while addressing unfinished business from the past.

- **Psychodynamic therapy:** Explores unconscious feelings and experiences from childhood that may influence current behavior.

- **Trauma-informed care:** Recognizes how past trauma impacts current life and focuses on creating safety and trust.

- **Mindfulness and meditation practices:** Help you become more aware of your inner child's emotions and needs, allowing for calm, compassionate responses.

Self-Care Practices for Healing

Healing your inner child also involves nurturing your emotional and creative self in ways that bring joy and comfort.

- **Journaling:** Writing can help you explore your inner child's emotions and past experiences.

- **Creative expression (art, music, writing):** Engaging in creative activities reconnects you with your playful, imaginative side.

- **Playfulness and leisure activities:** Doing things you enjoyed as a child—painting, dancing, or simply playing—can be healing.

- **Self-compassion exercises:** Learning to be kind and gentle with yourself, especially when you feel vulnerable, is crucial in healing.

- **Grounding techniques:** Deep breathing, meditation, or connecting with nature can help calm your inner child's emotional responses.

Books to Guide Your Healing Journey

There are numerous resources to support your journey:

- *Homecoming* by John Bradshaw: A powerful guide to reconnecting with your inner child.

- *The Inner Child Workbook* by Cathryn L. Taylor: A practical workbook for healing emotional wounds from childhood.

- *Healing the Shame That Binds You* by John Bradshaw: Focuses on overcoming the toxic shame often carried by the inner child.

Healing your inner child is a transformative journey that invites you to reconnect with the vulnerable parts of yourself that still carry childhood experiences. By acknowledging these emotions and offering yourself compassion, you can begin to heal past wounds and build a more fulfilling, peaceful life.

Remember, healing takes time—be gentle with yourself as you grow and nurture your inner child. The next chapter will provide practical tips for healing your inner child.

Chapter 7:

How Do I Heal My

Inner Child?

We nurture our creativity when we release our inner child. Let it run and roam free. It will take you on a brighter journey.
–Serina Hartwell

Have you ever noticed how certain situations trigger strong emotions, even when they seem unrelated to the present moment? These intense feelings may stem from unresolved childhood wounds carried by your inner child—the part of you that holds onto past emotions and experiences. As discussed in the previous chapter, healing your inner child involves reconnecting with these vulnerable parts of yourself and offering them the love and care they did not receive back then. This journey may feel daunting at first, but it is one of the most transformative steps toward emotional freedom, self-love, and inner peace.

In this chapter, we will guide you through the process of healing your inner child, from acknowledging its presence to reparenting yourself in a way that nurtures and supports your emotional well-being.

Step 1: Acknowledge and Accept

The first step in healing your inner child is acknowledging its presence and accepting the feelings and memories it holds. Many people spend their lives unconsciously avoiding or suppressing emotions tied to childhood, often because they are too painful to face. But ignoring these emotions does not make them disappear—they continue to influence your behavior and relationships in subtle yet powerful ways.

- **Recognize your inner child's presence:** Understand that your inner child is an integral part of you, representing your most vulnerable and emotional self. It is not something you outgrow or leave behind; it remains with you always.

- **Accept your inner child's feelings:** Whether you feel sadness, anger, fear, or even joy, it is important to accept these emotions as valid. Allow yourself to experience them fully rather than dismissing or pushing them away. This acceptance is where healing begins.

- **Understand the influence:** Your inner child shapes how you respond to stress, conflict, and relationships. By acknowledging its impact, you can identify patterns in your life that stem from unresolved childhood experiences.

For example, consider how you handle rejection. Suppose your inner child was wounded by a caregiver's emotional neglect. In that case, you may find yourself highly sensitive to any form of rejection in adulthood, reacting in ways that feel disproportionate to the current situation.

Step 2: Identify and Express Emotions

Once you've acknowledged your inner child, the next step is to identify and express the emotions tied to your childhood experiences. Often, these emotions have been repressed for years, but allowing them to surface is crucial to healing.

- **Journaling:** Writing about your childhood memories and emotions is a powerful way to explore your inner child's experiences. You might ask yourself, "What were my biggest fears as a child?" or "How did I feel when my needs were not met?" Allow yourself to write freely, without judgment.

- **Creative expression:** Art can facilitate healing when words are not enough. You might draw or paint images representing your inner child or use colors to express emotions. Creative expression allows your inner child to communicate in a non-verbal, intuitive way.

- **Talk to your inner child:** Some people find it helpful to write letters to their inner child or engage in internal dialogues. You might say, "I see you, I hear you, and I am here to take care of you now." This can create a sense of safety and acknowledgment.

- **Emotional release:** Healing your inner child often involves releasing emotions that have been bottled up for years. Crying, shouting, or even punching a pillow in a safe space can help you release anger, sadness, or frustration that has been trapped within you for too long.

Step 3: Reparenting

Reparenting is the act of becoming the caregiver your inner child needs. This step is essential because it allows you to fill the gaps left by your original caregivers, whether they were emotionally unavailable, critical, or neglectful.

- **Self-care:** Nurture yourself physically and emotionally, just as you would a child. Listen to your body's needs for rest, relaxation, and nourishment, while also tending to your emotional well-being.

- **Self-compassion:** Be kind to yourself, especially when you feel vulnerable. Practice speaking to yourself gently and understandingly, particularly when things do not go as planned. For example, if you make a mistake, replace harsh self-criticism with, "It is okay. I am learning, and I will do better next time."

- **Positive affirmations:** Replace the negative self-talk your inner child may have internalized with affirmations of love and worth. Statements like "I am worthy of love" or "I deserve care and attention" help rebuild your self-worth.

- **Boundary setting:** Learn to say "no" when necessary. Many of us grow up feeling that our needs do not matter, which can lead to poor boundaries in adulthood. Setting boundaries is a form of self-protection essential to reparenting your inner child.

Step 4: Reframe Negative Experiences

Healing does not mean erasing the past; it involves reframing it in a way that allows for growth and resilience. How you perceive your childhood experiences can shape how you feel about yourself today.

- **Reframe traumatic experiences:** Rather than seeing yourself solely as a victim, try to identify lessons or strengths that emerged from those experiences. This is not about excusing what happened but shifting from powerlessness to empowerment. For example, you might say, "I survived that, and it made me stronger."

- **Challenge negative self-talk:** If your inner child believes messages like "I am not good enough" or "I do not deserve love," it is time to question these thoughts. Ask yourself, "Is this belief really true?" Then replace it with positive, realistic affirmations that support your self-worth.

- **Practice forgiveness:** Forgiveness can be one of the hardest steps, especially if your childhood was marked by neglect or abuse. Forgiving does not mean forgetting or excusing—it means releasing the hold that anger and resentment have on you. Forgiveness is for your peace, allowing you to move forward without carrying the burden of past hurt.

Step 5: Integrate Your Inner Child

The final step in healing is to integrate your inner child into your adult self, developing a balanced relationship where your inner child's needs are acknowledged without overwhelming your life.

- **Mindfulness:** Practice being present with your inner child's emotions as they arise. When you notice an emotional trigger, take a moment to pause, breathe, and recognize it as your inner child seeking attention. Mindfulness allows you to respond thoughtfully rather than react impulsively.

- **Grounding techniques:** When your inner child feels overwhelmed, grounding exercises can calm your nervous system. Deep breathing, meditation, or connecting with nature can bring you back to the present moment, helping you manage intense emotions more effectively.

- **Self-awareness:** Over time, you will become more attuned to your inner child's triggers and patterns. This awareness enables you to navigate relationships, stress, and challenges with greater understanding and emotional balance.

Additional Techniques for Healing

While the foundational steps form the core of inner child healing, these additional techniques can help deepen the process.

- **Meditation and visualization:** Guided meditations that focus on connecting with your inner child can help you access repressed emotions and memories in a safe space. Visualizing your younger self can evoke compassion and healing energy.

- **Inner child dialogues:** Similar to journaling, engaging in conversations with your inner child can help you understand its needs and fears. Speaking directly to this part of yourself builds trust and fosters emotional safety.

- **Creative therapies:** Art, music, and drama can unlock emotions and memories that may be hard to access through words alone. These therapies allow your inner child to express itself freely.

- **Somatic experiencing:** This trauma release technique helps process unresolved trauma stored in the body. Focusing on physical sensations can release trapped energy and emotions, allowing your nervous system to regulate.

- **EMDR (Eye Movement Desensitization and Reprocessing):** EMDR is a trauma therapy that uses eye movements to help process and heal from traumatic experiences. It is particularly effective for individuals whose inner child holds deep trauma.

Do Not Hesitate to Seek Support

Healing your inner child can be challenging, and seeking support when needed is essential. Many resources and professionals can guide you through this journey.

- **Therapists or counselors:** Look for a therapist who specializes in inner child work or trauma. They can offer guidance, emotional support, and techniques tailored to your specific needs.

- **Support groups or online forums:** Connecting with others on similar journeys can be incredibly healing. Sharing experiences, challenges, and successes within a supportive community helps you feel less alone.

- **Trusted friends or family members:** Opening up to people you trust about your inner child healing can provide accountability and emotional support. Just make sure they are individuals who understand and respect your process.

Healing your inner child is a transformative journey that can lead to emotional freedom, self-compassion, and healthier relationships. By accepting your inner child, expressing repressed emotions, and reparenting yourself with love and care, you can break free from old patterns.

In the next chapter, we will explore how healing your inner child can help you attract healthier relationships filled with love and compassion.

Chapter 8:

Why Does Healing Your Inner Child Result in Attracting Healthier Relationships?

When you feel a child inside of you springing to life, that's how you know you're where you should be. –C. JoyBell C

Ever wonder why you keep finding yourself in the same kind of unhealthy relationships? The answer might lie deep within—inside your inner child. Healing your inner child does not just address childhood wounds; it transforms how you see yourself and your relationships. By nurturing this vulnerable part of yourself, you cultivate self-love, self-worth, and emotional resilience—all essential for attracting healthier, more fulfilling relationships.

Imagine what happens when you start loving yourself unconditionally, setting clear boundaries, and managing your emotions with maturity. You begin to attract partners who value and respect you, rather than those who reflect old, toxic patterns from the past. Healing your inner child rewrites the emotional script you have been following, freeing you from cycles of unhealthy relationships.

This chapter will explore how this inner transformation leads to better relationship dynamics and helps you create the love and connection you deserve. Keep reading to discover how nurturing your inner child paves the way for deeper, healthier relationships with others—and, most importantly, with yourself.

How Inner Healing Reflects on the Outside

Healing your inner child transforms how you relate to yourself and others. As you cultivate self-love and self-acceptance, your relationships begin to reflect this inner transformation. You no longer feel the need to seek validation from others or tolerate disrespect because your sense of worth comes from within.

- **Self-love and self-acceptance:** When you love and accept yourself, you naturally attract partners who respect and value you. You stop settling for people who do not treat you well because you recognize your inherent worth. For example, someone who once clung to emotionally unavailable partners may find themselves drawn to nurturing, attentive individuals simply because their self-worth has grown.

- **Emotional regulation:** Healing your inner child teaches you how to manage your emotions effectively. Instead of reacting impulsively or shutting down during conflict, you learn to pause, reflect, and respond thoughtfully. This emotional maturity allows for smoother conflict resolution, reducing misunderstandings and drama in relationships.

- **Clear boundaries:** A healed inner child understands the importance of setting and maintaining healthy boundaries. When you know your worth, you are not afraid to communicate your needs and expectations. Boundaries become a means of protecting your emotional health rather than a source of conflict.

- **Self-worth:** One of the most transformative effects of inner child healing is a newfound sense of self-worth. You are less likely to settle for toxic or abusive relationships because you know what you deserve. Instead of seeking love from those who cannot give it, you focus on nurturing your own well-being.

Healthy Relationship Patterns

Once you have healed your inner child, you will begin to attract and cultivate healthy relationship patterns. These patterns are grounded in mutual respect, emotional maturity, and open communication—essential components for lasting and fulfilling relationships.

- **Secure attachment style:** Healing your inner child helps you develop a secure attachment style, where you feel safe being emotionally vulnerable and trusting in relationships. You are no longer afraid of closeness, nor do you push people away out of fear of being hurt. Instead, you form deep, trusting connections with others who are also emotionally available.

- **Emotional maturity:** Emotional maturity is key to maintaining healthy relationships. Once you have healed your inner child, you are better equipped to handle conflicts and emotions responsibly. You no longer lash out or shut down when challenges arise. Instead, you address issues calmly and empathetically, fostering stronger, more resilient relationships.

- **Effective communication:** Clear, honest communication is a hallmark of healthy relationships. A healed inner child empowers you to express your needs, desires, and feelings openly, without the fear of rejection or judgment. You no longer feel the need to hide your emotions or pretend to be someone you are not to please others.

- **Mutual respect:** As you heal, you attract partners who respect your boundaries, feelings, and autonomy. Healthy relationships are built on mutual respect, where each partner values the other's individuality and emotional needs. For example, if you have always struggled to ask for emotional support in relationships, healing your inner child can empower you to communicate your needs more confidently. You will attract partners who are willing to listen and offer the care and support you deserve.

No Longer Attracting Toxic Partners

One of the most powerful benefits of healing your inner child is breaking free from toxic relationship patterns. Many of us unconsciously repeat unhealthy dynamics because they feel familiar, even though they are harmful. When you heal your inner child, you gain the awareness and strength to choose healthier relationships.

- **Break free from toxic patterns:** Healing allows you to recognize the red flags of unhealthy relationships early on, so you no longer fall into the same traps. You become more attuned to what a healthy relationship looks like and begin avoiding partners who display toxic behaviors, such as manipulation, emotional unavailability, or disrespect.

- **No longer seeking validation:** In the past, you may have sought validation from your partners, believing their approval would make you feel whole. After healing, you no longer depend on others for a sense of self-worth. You become secure in yourself, making you less likely to stay in a relationship simply for validation.

- **Empowered decision-making:** Healing your inner child enables you to make decisions that align with your values and emotional well-being. Rather than choosing partners out of fear or insecurity, you make these choices from a place of empowerment. You are no longer afraid to walk away from relationships that do not serve you because you trust yourself to make the right decisions. For instance, someone who once stayed in toxic relationships out of fear of being alone might, after healing, feel confident enough to end those relationships and choose partners who align with their growth and happiness.

Attracting Nurturing Partners

As you heal, you begin to attract partners who reflect the nurturing, supportive energy you have cultivated within yourself. Healthy relationships become a natural extension of the love and care you provide for yourself.

- **Self-care and self-love:** The more you practice self-care and self-love, the more you attract partners who support and nurture you. Healthy relationships are built on the foundation of mutual care, where both partners encourage each other's growth and well-being.

- **Emotional intelligence:** Healing your inner child enhances your emotional intelligence, allowing you to recognize and appreciate emotional intelligence in others. You are drawn to partners who are self-aware, empathetic, and capable of forming deep emotional connections.

- **Healthy vulnerability:** After healing, you become more open to healthy vulnerability. You are no longer afraid to let others see the real you, and you attract partners who are equally open and willing to be vulnerable. This creates a deeper emotional connection and allows authentic love to flourish. For example, someone who used to build emotional walls in relationships might now be able to open up and be vulnerable with a partner who respects their feelings, fostering a more nurturing and supportive connection.

Signs of Healing Your Inner Child

As you progress on your healing journey, you will begin to notice signs that indicate you are on the right path. These signs reflect the inner work you are doing and the positive changes that are unfolding in your relationships.

- **Increased self-awareness:** You become more aware of your emotional triggers and how to manage them. Rather than reacting impulsively, you take the time to understand the source of your emotions and respond mindfully.

- **Improved emotional regulation:** You can regulate your emotions more effectively, even in difficult situations. This allows you to navigate conflicts in relationships with calmness and clarity, rather than escalating into emotional outbursts or withdrawing.

- **Healthier boundaries:** You establish and maintain healthier boundaries, recognizing that setting limits is an act of self-love. You no longer feel guilty for saying "no" when something does not align with your emotional well-being.

- **Enhanced self-compassion:** You treat yourself with more kindness and understanding, especially during challenging times. You no longer engage in harsh self-criticism or self-blame, and you extend the same compassion to others.

- **More fulfilling relationships:** Your inner healing leads to more fulfilling relationships. You attract people who respect, love, and support you in healthy ways, allowing you to build deeper emotional connections with them.

Relationship Benefits of Healing Your Inner Child

Healing your inner child brings many benefits to your relationships, enhancing romantic partnerships, family dynamics, and professional connections. These positive changes can transform the way you relate to others.

- **Deeper emotional connections:** Healing allows you to form more personal and intimate connections with others. You are no longer afraid of intimacy or vulnerability, allowing yourself to experience these relationships in their truest form.

- **Improved communication:** Clear, honest communication becomes a natural part of your relationships. You can express yourself and your feelings openly, leading to greater understanding and fewer misunderstandings.

- **Increased intimacy:** Healing your inner child fosters greater emotional and physical intimacy. You become more comfortable with closeness, deepening your bond with your partner.

- **Healthier conflict resolution:** You will be better equipped to resolve conflicts in healthy and respectful ways. With improved emotional regulation and communication skills, you no longer avoid issues or escalate arguments. Instead, you approach challenges with empathy and understanding.

- **Mutual growth and support:** Healthy relationships create a space for mutual growth and support. Both you and your partner are committed to each other's well-being, encouraging each other to grow and evolve together.

By nurturing the vulnerable parts of yourself, setting boundaries, communicating openly, and loving yourself unconditionally, you will naturally attract partners who reflect this same energy. Remember, healing is a journey that requires patience, self-compassion, and awareness. As you continue this process, you will cultivate the love and connection you truly deserve in all areas of your life.

The next chapter will offer practical tips on finding love while healing.

Chapter 9:

Finding Love Throughout Your Healing Journey

The wound is where the light enters you. –Rumi

Finding love while healing is both a challenge and a gift. When you have experienced emotional wounds, it is easy to believe that love will elude you until you are "fully healed." But healing is a lifelong process, and love can still find you. During your healing journey, you become more open to discovering love that is deeper, more genuine, and built on mutual growth. Learning to love and be loved while healing allows you to experience relationships with newfound awareness and self-compassion.

This chapter focuses on how to find love while nurturing yourself. You will discover that embracing vulnerability, navigating relationships with care, and prioritizing self-love are essential parts of this journey. You will also learn that the love you give and receive during this time can be transformative, helping you grow as a person and build more meaningful connections. Whether you are just beginning your healing process or have been on this path for some time, this chapter will guide you in balancing personal growth with the openness needed to cultivate real love.

Embracing Vulnerability

As you heal, you will naturally reflect on past experiences and how they have shaped who you are today. Healing is not about reaching perfection but about embracing your imperfections and striving to become the best version of yourself. Through self-reflection, you can recognize patterns that no longer serve you and make intentional changes. For example, if you have always been afraid of intimacy due to past hurts, healing offers you the opportunity to explore that fear and learn how to approach love in a new way.

Finding love during your healing journey requires a willingness to be vulnerable. Vulnerability is not about oversharing or putting yourself at risk; it is about being honest with your emotions and allowing others to see the real you. When you open up, you create space for authentic connection. It might feel risky to expose your feelings, especially after experiencing past pain, but vulnerability is the key to forming meaningful relationships.

As you embrace vulnerability, you will seek relationships grounded in trust, empathy, and mutual support—connections that encourage growth. These relationships are built on the understanding that neither partner is perfect, but both are committed to showing up for one another, even during difficult times. Love in these relationships is not transactional; it is a shared journey of mutual care, understanding, and growth.

Navigating Relationships

When you are healing, it is important not to rush into relationships. Sometimes, the desire to fill emotional voids can lead you to seek love before you are truly ready. Allow yourself the time to heal at your own pace. It is perfectly okay to take a step back, reflect, and build a relationship slowly. Healing is not a race, and neither is love. For example, if you have just emerged from a difficult relationship, give yourself the space to process those emotions before jumping into something new.

One of the most powerful tools you gain during your healing journey is the ability to set and maintain healthy boundaries. Boundaries are essential for protecting your emotional well-being and ensuring that your relationships are balanced. Whether it is saying "no" to things that drain your energy or clearly communicating what you need from a partner, boundaries allow you to engage in relationships from a place of strength rather than insecurity. By setting clear limits, you demonstrate that your emotional health matters, which in turn attracts partners who respect those boundaries.

Effective communication is the backbone of any healthy relationship, especially when healing. It is crucial to be honest with your partner about where you are emotionally and what you need. Transparent communication builds trust and ensures that you and your partner are on the same page. For instance, you might say, "I am working through some personal issues and may need extra time to process my feelings." Being upfront about your emotional state fosters understanding and strengthens the bond between you and your partner.

Mindset Shifts

Your thoughts shape your reality, so focusing on empowering beliefs during your healing journey is essential. Positive affirmations can help shift your mindset from self-doubt to self-empowerment. By repeating affirmations like "I am worthy of love" or "I deserve healthy relationships," you begin to internalize these beliefs, gradually making them a reality. Over time, this shift in mindset makes you more open to attracting love that aligns with your true worth.

Practicing gratitude is another powerful mindset shift. When you focus on what you are grateful for, you cultivate a sense of abundance rather than scarcity. Gratitude helps you appreciate the beauty in life and relationships, even when things are not perfect. By focusing on what is going well, you open yourself up to more positive experiences and attract relationships that reflect that same energy. For instance, rather than dwelling on what is missing in a relationship, you might choose to focus on how your partner shows care and affection.

Healing is not a linear process—it comes with setbacks and challenges. Developing resilience allows you to cope with life's ups and downs without losing hope. When you build resilience, you learn to see challenges as opportunities for growth rather than obstacles. This mindset shift is especially helpful in relationships, where resilience helps you navigate conflicts without fear or defensiveness. Instead of giving up when things get tough, resilience helps you work through issues and come out stronger on the other side.

Spiritual Connection

Healing your inner child and finding love often involve seeking inner peace. This peace does not come from external validation but from a deep connection with yourself and the world around you. When you find this peace, you become more present in your relationships and approach love with a calm, open heart. You become less reactive and more grounded, allowing you to enjoy the journey rather than constantly worrying about the destination.

Mindfulness is another key practice in this process. It encourages you to live fully in the present moment, embracing life as it is rather than getting caught up in the past or future. In relationships, mindfulness helps you appreciate your partner for who they truly are, not who you expect them to be. It allows you to experience love more fully, free from the anxieties that often arise from overthinking or worrying about what comes next.

For some, spirituality or faith can play a significant role in the healing journey. Whether you believe in a higher power, the universe, or a greater sense of purpose, connecting to something bigger than yourself can provide guidance and strength. It helps you find meaning in your experiences, trust the healing process, and feel supported as you navigate personal growth and relationships.

Finding love throughout your healing journey is an exciting experience. As you heal, you become more open to the love that aligns with your true self and builds relationships based on mutual respect and emotional maturity. Remember, your most important relationship is with yourself—nurture it, and the rest will follow.

The next chapter will explore why loving yourself should always be your highest priority.

Chapter 10:

Loving Yourself Will Always Need to Be Your Highest Priority

Our sorrows and wounds are healed only when we touch them with compassion. –Jack Kornfield

Imagine a life where you consistently show up for yourself with kindness, forgive your mistakes and celebrate your successes. Imagine how self-love could transform your relationships, career, and overall well-being. Loving yourself is not about being self-centered or egotistical; it is about nurturing the foundation of who you are. Without self-love, we may rely on external validation, constantly seek approval, and struggle to set boundaries. But when you prioritize loving yourself, you unlock a life filled with confidence, resilience, and fulfillment.

This chapter will explore why self-love is the foundation of a happy and successful life. We will discuss how embracing self-compassion, setting boundaries, and practicing mindfulness can lead to healthier relationships, a stronger sense of self, and inner peace. Self-love does not just happen overnight; it is a continuous practice that evolves as you grow. By prioritizing yourself, you create a ripple effect that touches every aspect of your life. Read on!

Self-Love Foundations

Here are some foundational aspects of self-love to understand:

1. Self-Acceptance

Self-love begins with self-acceptance, which means embracing every part of who you are—your strengths, weaknesses, and even the parts of yourself you wish were different. Self-acceptance is about acknowledging your imperfections without letting them define your worth. It is understanding that you are whole, even with flaws. For example, instead of criticizing yourself for not being as outgoing as others, you might appreciate your introspective, thoughtful nature. Self-acceptance allows you to live authentically without constantly striving to meet unrealistic standards set by others.

2. Self-Compassion

Treating yourself with compassion is another cornerstone of self-love. Just as you would comfort a friend in hard times, self-compassion is about offering yourself the same kindness, understanding, and patience. When you make a mistake or fall short of your goals, self-compassion encourages you to respond with grace rather than harsh judgment. It is about recognizing that everyone struggles and being kind to yourself during those moments. For instance, if you do not get the job you applied for, instead of berating yourself, you might say, "It is okay. I did my best, and I will keep trying. Sometimes things do not work out because something better is ahead." This shift in perspective builds resilience and helps you maintain a positive outlook.

3. Self-Forgiveness

We often hold onto guilt and regret, replaying our past mistakes and letting them undermine our self-worth. Self-love requires self-forgiveness, which means releasing the self-criticism and guilt that keep you stuck. Forgiveness does not excuse harmful behavior; it allows you to let go of the emotional weight these experiences carry. By forgiving yourself, you free up mental and emotional space for growth and healing. For example, if you have made mistakes in past relationships, self-forgiveness allows you to learn from those experiences without punishing yourself indefinitely.

Benefits of Self-Love

Self-love is the foundation of emotional well-being, allowing you to embrace your true self without relying on external validation. Here are some of its key benefits:

1. **Confidence**

One of the immediate benefits of self-love is increased confidence. When you love yourself, you develop a positive self-image and assertiveness, allowing you to take up space in the world without hesitation. Confidence rooted in self-love is not about being boastful; it is about knowing your worth and standing firm in your values. You begin to trust your decisions and feel empowered to pursue your goals without fear of failure. For example, someone who practices self-love may feel more confident asking for a raise at work or setting boundaries in relationships.

2. **Resilience**

Life is full of challenges, but self-love equips you with the resilience to navigate setbacks. Loving yourself helps you bounce back from adversity because you believe in your ability to overcome difficulties. Resilience does not mean avoiding hardship; it means facing challenges with the understanding that you are strong enough to handle them. With self-love, you can keep going even when things go wrong. For instance, after experiencing a personal loss, someone with strong self-love may allow themselves to grieve but also find ways to heal and move forward.

3. **Healthy Relationships**

Self-love is the foundation of all healthy relationships. When you love yourself, you set the standard for how others should treat you, refusing to tolerate disrespect or manipulation. Healthy relationships are built on mutual respect, and practicing self-love attracts people who honor your boundaries and support your growth. For example, rather than remaining in a toxic friendship that constantly drains you, self-love might encourage you to seek connections that uplift and energize you.

Practices for Self-Love

Practicing self-love involves intentional habits that nurture your mental, emotional, and physical well-being. These practices help you cultivate a healthier relationship with yourself, promoting inner peace and self-acceptance.

1. **Self-Care**

Self-care is one of the most tangible ways to practice self-love. It is more than bubble baths and spa days—self-care means prioritizing your physical, emotional, and mental well-being. This could be as simple as taking a walk when you feel stressed, eating nourishing meals, or setting aside time to relax. Self-care involves making choices that support your overall health and happiness, even when life gets busy. For example, taking a mental health day when you are feeling overwhelmed is a form of self-care that honors your need for rest and rejuvenation.

2. **Boundary Setting**

Boundaries are essential for protecting your emotional well-being, and setting them is a powerful act of self-love. Establishing healthy boundaries creates limits that define what is acceptable in your relationships and interactions, allowing you to protect your energy and prioritize your needs without guilt. For instance, saying "no" to additional work when you are already overwhelmed is a way to set a boundary that safeguards your mental health. By setting boundaries, you teach others to treat you with respect and care.

Overcoming Obstacles

Overcoming obstacles requires resilience and a growth-oriented mindset, even in the face of challenges. Here are some tips for overcoming common obstacles to self-love:

1. Self-Criticism

One of the biggest obstacles to self-love is self-criticism. Many of us have an inner critic constantly pointing out our flaws, mistakes, or shortcomings. To overcome self-criticism, it is essential to challenge these negative thoughts and reframe them more compassionately. For example, if your inner critic says, "I am not good enough," try countering that thought with, "I am doing my best, and that is enough." By consistently challenging negative self-talk, you can weaken its influence and replace it with more supportive, uplifting beliefs.

2. Trauma and Past Hurts

Healing from trauma and past hurts is a crucial part of the self-love journey. Trauma can leave emotional scars that make it difficult to feel worthy of love, but by seeking support and working through your pain, you can begin to let go of what holds you back. Therapy, support groups, and other healing practices can help you process unresolved emotions and reclaim your self-worth. For example, someone who experienced childhood neglect may need to work through feelings of abandonment to fully embrace self-love.

3. Societal Pressure

We are constantly bombarded with messages about how we should look, act, or live, making it easy to fall into the comparison trap. Society often sets unrealistic expectations that can leave us feeling inadequate or unworthy. Overcoming societal pressure means learning to ignore those external voices and focusing on what truly matters to you. For instance, rather than striving for a "perfect" body due to societal standards, you might focus on feeling healthy and strong, regardless of appearance. Remember, self-love is about living authentically, not about meeting others' expectations.

Empowerment Through Self-Love

Empowerment through self-love comes from recognizing your worth and embracing your strengths.

By prioritizing your well-being, you build the confidence to take control of your life and make choices that align with your true values.

1. **Autonomy**

Self-love fosters a greater sense of autonomy, allowing you to make decisions that align with your values and needs without being swayed by external pressures. When you trust yourself, you feel empowered to take control of your life. For example, if you are deciding whether to accept a new job, self-love might encourage you to choose the path that brings joy and fulfillment rather than one that looks good on paper but does not resonate with your true desires.

2. **Authenticity**

Loving yourself helps you live authentically, embracing your true self without fear of judgment. When you are comfortable in your own skin, you are more likely to express your thoughts, feelings, and desires openly, without trying to fit into someone else's mold. Authenticity means showing up as you are—flaws and all—and trusting that you are enough. For example, instead of pretending to be more outgoing to fit in with a particular group, you might embrace your introverted nature and seek friendships that appreciate and respect who you truly are.

3. **Inner Peace**

One of the greatest gifts of self-love is inner peace. Inner peace comes from knowing that you are enough just as you are and that your worth is not dependent on external factors like achievements or relationships. Cultivating self-love fosters a deep contentment that life's ups and downs cannot shake. For instance, even when faced with challenges or criticism, self-love helps you stay grounded in the knowledge that you are worthy, loved, and deserving of happiness. This inner peace gives you the calm confidence to move through life's changes with resilience, unaffected by outside chaos.

Loving yourself should always be a top priority because it forms the foundation for a happy, fulfilling life. When you cultivate self-love, you build resilience, attract healthier relationships, and experience inner peace. Remember, self-love is not a destination; it is a lifelong journey that requires compassion, patience, and commitment. By prioritizing yourself, you create the life you truly deserve.

In the next chapter, we will explore practical tips for raising a child to stay connected to their inner self.

Chapter 11

How to Raise Your Children so They Stay Connected With Their Inner Child and Learn to Nurture and Heal Themselves From a Young Age

If we don't shape our kids, they will be shaped by outside forces that don't care what shape our kids are in. –Dr. Louise Hart

Becoming a mother has been the most transformative experience of my life. For the first time, I have felt true, unconditional love—not just for my daughter, but for myself as well. In raising her, I have learned so much about patience, forgiveness, and healing—things I wish I had known as a child. I have realized how essential it is to create an environment where children feel safe, can freely express their emotions, and do not have to bear the weight of unhealed traumas from generations before them. Watching my daughter thrive, unburdened by the pain I once carried, fills me with hope and pride. As I continue to heal my inner child, I understand how important it is to raise children in a way that keeps them connected to theirs.

This chapter is for every parent who wants to help their children grow up emotionally healthy and whole. It is for those who want to break cycles of trauma and raise children who can nurture and heal themselves from a young age. Raising children this way is not just about providing love and care; it is about creating a foundation where they are free to be themselves and learn to face life's challenges with resilience and self-compassion. By helping our children stay connected to their inner child, we teach them to protect their emotional well-being, even in a world that may try to tear them down.

Building a Foundation for Emotional Safety

One of the most important things you can do for your child is to create a space where they feel emotionally safe. This goes beyond just providing physical security; it means making sure they feel heard, understood, and valued. As a child, I never felt safe enough to share my emotions with my parents. Whenever I tried, I felt dismissed or, worse, criticized. As a result, I learned to bottle up my feelings, which only led to more pain over time.

With my daughter, I have made it a priority to ensure she knows she can talk to me about anything without fear of judgment. She understands that her feelings are valid—whether she is upset about how someone treats her or anxious about a new challenge. I have shown her that her emotions matter by listening without immediately trying to fix things or telling her what to do. Because she feels safe to express herself, she is more likely to stay connected to her inner child—the part of her that holds her deepest emotions and desires.

How to Create Emotional Safety

Creating emotional safety for your child is essential for fostering trust and open communication. Here are some ways to help:

- **Listen without judgment:** When your child shares their feelings, resist the urge to correct or dismiss them. Allow them to express themselves fully before offering advice, showing that you respect their emotions.

- **Validate their emotions:** Even if their feelings seem small or irrational to you, remember that these emotions are significant to them. Use phrases like, "I understand why you feel this way" or "It is okay to feel sad."

- **Be available:** Make sure your child knows you are there to talk; no matter how busy life gets. Whether they are upset or simply excited to share something, being present helps build trust and reinforces their sense of safety.

Teaching Self-Compassion From a Young Age

One of the greatest gifts we can give our children is the ability to be kind to themselves. As adults, many of us struggle with self-criticism, a habit often ingrained in childhood. I remember constantly feeling like I was not enough—smart enough, pretty enough, good enough. These feelings came from external pressures and the way I was taught to view myself. I was never taught self-compassion, and I have had to learn it the hard way through my healing journey.

With my daughter, I have made it a point to teach her that mistakes are a natural part of life. Instead of criticizing herself when she messes up, I encourage her to be kind to herself and understand that she is still learning and growing. When she struggles with how to respond when another child is mean to her or feels disappointed after a figure skating competition, I encourage her to adopt a growth mindset. I remind her that often, people act out because they are struggling with their own issues. Next time, she may find a new way to interact with them or simply remove herself from those interactions. But no matter what, I remind her not to let that negative experience define her. I tell her, "You did your best, and that is enough." By nurturing self-compassion and teaching her to understand others' behavior, I hope to give her the strength to face life's challenges with resilience rather than self-doubt.

Ways to Teach Self-Compassion

Here are some ways to teach your child self-compassion:

- **Model self-kindness:** Children learn by watching us. When you make a mistake, show your child how to be gentle with yourself. Instead of saying, "I am so stupid for doing that," say, "I made a mistake, but it is okay. I will learn from it."

- **Encourage positive self-talk:** Help your child develop a habit of speaking kindly to themselves. When they say something negative like, "I am not good at this," encourage them to reframe it: "I am still learning, and I am getting better every day."

- **Celebrate effort, not just results:** Focus on the hard work your child puts into something rather than just the outcome. This helps them value their effort and progress instead of tying their worth solely to success.

The Power of Play and Creativity

One of the most direct ways to help children stay connected to their inner child is through play and creativity. Children are naturally imaginative, and allowing them to explore this creativity helps them stay in touch with their curiosity, wonder, and joy. As adults, we often lose sight of the importance of play, becoming too focused on responsibilities and productivity. However, for children, play is essential for emotional development and healing.

I encourage my daughter to engage in activities that allow her to express herself creatively—whether it is playing an instrument, painting, or simply playing pretend. These moments of play help her stay connected to her inner child, enabling her to explore her emotions and the world around her in a safe and joyful way.

Ways to Encourage Creativity and Play

Here are some ways to encourage creativity and play in your child:

- **Provide creative outlets:** Whether it is art supplies, musical instruments, or a designated play space, give your child the tools they need to explore their creativity.

- **Join them in play:** Spend time playing with your child, whether it is building with blocks or creating stories together. This strengthens your bond and shows them that play is valuable at any age.

- **Celebrate their creativity:** When your child creates something—whether it is a drawing or a new song—celebrate it with them. This reinforces the idea that their creativity is important and valued.

Raising a child who stays connected to their inner child and learns to nurture and heal themselves from a young age is one of the greatest gifts you can give. It is about creating a foundation of emotional safety, teaching self-compassion, setting boundaries, and encouraging emotional expression and creativity. As parents, we have the power to break cycles of trauma and raise emotionally whole children.

Final Thoughts

Healing from childhood trauma and narcissistic abuse is a journey that can feel lonely, overwhelming, and at times, nearly impossible. Yet here you are, at the end of this book, having explored some of the deepest, most vulnerable parts of yourself. You have faced pain that may have remained unspoken for years, found compassion for the parts of yourself that have been hurting, and taken steps toward self-acceptance and self-love. This is not the end of your journey—healing is a lifelong commitment. But reaching this point speaks to your resilience, courage, and readiness to reclaim your life from the pain of the past.

A key step in this journey has been understanding narcissistic abuse and how its impact infiltrates every part of our lives. Those who have endured it know the scars it leaves: the self-doubt, the constant feeling of being "not enough," and the fear of never truly being seen or valued. By exploring these patterns, you have gained clarity that releases you from self-blame. This knowledge reveals that the cycles of manipulation and control you experienced were never reflections of your worth. With this understanding, you can finally start letting go of any guilt or shame you have carried, knowing that the actions of others are not your fault.

As you moved through the chapters on attachment styles and codependency, you may have recognized yourself in some of the descriptions. Perhaps you saw patterns that have held you back or led to relationships that left you feeling depleted. These behaviors often stem from early childhood experiences with caregivers, shaping the way we connect with others as adults. Exploring your attachment style can be eye-opening, revealing how past experiences have influenced your views on love, intimacy, and self-worth. Recognizing these patterns is not easy, but it is incredibly empowering—you are no longer bound to repeat them. By understanding how your attachment style has influenced your relationships, you now have the tools to make different choices, ones that honor who you are today and what you truly deserve.

Self-love may have been one of the hardest concepts to embrace. For many, self-love is unfamiliar territory, especially if you have spent years believing your worth depended on others' opinions. When you have been conditioned to seek validation outside yourself, it can feel impossible to turn inward for acceptance. Yet, loving yourself—your whole self, including the parts that feel flawed or damaged—is the foundation of true healing. Self-love is not about perfection; it is about embracing yourself as you are. It means choosing to respect, nurture, and uplift yourself daily, even when it is hard. As you continue this journey, remember that self-love is the cornerstone of all healthy relationships and personal growth.

For parents, this book also highlighted the importance of raising children in a way that allows them to stay connected to their own inner child. Creating a safe, loving environment where children are free to express their emotions without fear of judgment is one of the most powerful ways to break cycles of trauma. By fostering self-compassion, empathy, and open communication, you give your children tools that many of us had to learn much later in life. Showing them that their emotions matter and that they are loved and valued creates a foundation of self-worth that will support them throughout their lives. You are giving your children what you may not have received, and that is an incredible act of love.

In the later chapters, the focus shifted toward how healing your inner child naturally leads to healthier relationships. When you prioritize your emotional needs and cultivate self-love, you are no longer drawn to relationships that drain you. Instead, you begin to attract relationships that reflect the respect, empathy, and kindness you have started showing yourself. This does not mean you will never face challenges, but it does mean you will have the resilience and self-respect to navigate them with strength. Healthy relationships are built on mutual support, where both partners feel safe to express their true selves. By healing yourself, you open the door to connections that honor who you are and celebrate your growth.

Healing from narcissistic abuse and reconnecting with your inner child is not something that happens overnight. It is a lifelong commitment to caring for yourself, choosing to love yourself when it feels impossible, and releasing beliefs that no longer serve you. Healing is not linear—there will be setbacks, moments of doubt, and times when old wounds resurface. But with each step forward, you reclaim more of your strength, peace, and right to happiness. Healing is not about erasing the past but about creating a future where you can live free from its shadows.

You have made remarkable progress, and good things lie ahead for you. Keep moving forward with bravery, patience, and kindness toward yourself. Healing takes time, and every step you take is a testament to your strength. The life you deserve—one filled with acceptance, happiness, and love—is within reach. Believe in yourself, because you are worth it.

References

Attachment styles & their role in our adult relationships. (2020, July 2). Attachment Project. https://www.attachmentproject.com/blog/four-attachment-styles/

Baulch, D. J. (2023, October 24). *What is inner child work and how do you get started?* Inner Melbourne Psychology. https://www.innermelbpsychology.com.au/what-is-inner-child-work-and-how-to-get-started/

Best 50 attachment styles quotes. (n.d.). Ineffable Living. https://ineffableliving.com/best-attachment-styles-quotes/

Big Nehe (Content Guru). (2024, April 25). *21 narcissistic abuse healing quotes.* Medium. https://nehemiahisamotu.medium.com/21-narcissistic-abuse-healing-quotes-783eb5cb66f0

Boudin, M. (2023, May 30). *11 quotes about narcissism from actual therapists.* Choosing Therapy. https://www.choosingtherapy.com/narcissist-quotes/

Brennan, D. (2023, March 30). *Narcissism: Symptoms and signs.* WebMD. https://www.webmd.com/mental-health/narcissism-symptoms-signs

Codependent no more quotes by Melody Beattie. (n.d.). https://www.goodreads.com/work/quotes/70 6540-codependent-no-more-how-to-stop-controlling-others-and-start-caring-for

Cooks-Campbell, A. (2022, March 15). *How inner child work enables healing and playful discovery.* BetterUp. https://www.betterup.com/blog/inner-child-work

Dodgson, L. (2018, January 23). *Why empaths and narcissists are attracted to each other.* Business Insider. https://www.businessinsider.com/why-empaths-and-narcissists-are-attracted-to-each-other-2018-1?r=US&IR=T

Fargo, S. (n.d.). *60 healing quotes that inspire: A journey to inner peace.* Mindfulness Exercises. https://mindfulnessexercises.com/healing-quotes/

Gould, W. R. (2020, May 21). *What is codependency?* Verywell Mind. https://www.verywellmind.com/what-is-codependency-5072124

Mandriota, M. (2021, October 13). *4 types of attachment: What's your style?* Psych Central. https://psychcentral.com/health/4-attachment-styles-in-relationships

Mental Health America. (2023). *Co-dependency*. Mental Health America. https://www.mhanational.org/co-dependency

Morin, A. (2024, June 6). *These 23 parenting quotes will help you keep calm, cool, and collected*. Parents. https://www.parents.com/inspirational-parenting-quotes-8654013

Narcissistic personality disorder. (2023, April 6). Mayo Clinic. https://www.mayoclinic.org/diseases-conditions/narcissistic-personality-disorder/symptoms-causes/syc-20366662

Neurharth, D. (2017, August 15). *25 spot-on quotations about narcissism*. Psych Central. https://psychcentral.com/blog/narcissism-decoded/2017/08/25-spot-on-quotations-about-narcissism

Parker, A. (2023, February 13). *How I break free from anxious to secure attachment style*. Medium. https://medium.com/@ohanusiebuka21/how-i-break-free-from-anxious-to-secure-attachment-style-18ed619e8705

Purkayastha, R. (2022, November 17). *9 inner child quotes that will make you come alive*. Medium. https://medium.com/@mail2rajashree/9-inner-child-quotes-that-will-make-you-come-alive-3f7fa03cc2b4

Saxena, S. (2023, September 5). *The dangerous relationship between empaths & narcissists*. Choosing Therapy. https://www.choosingtherapy.com/empaths-and-narcissists/